To the Land of the Lost
Saving My Child from the Grip of Asperger's

Tracy M. Maguire

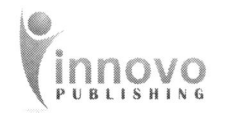

innovo
PUBLISHING

Published by
Innovo Publishing, LLC
www.innovopublishing.com
1-888-546-2111

Providing Full-Service Publishing Services for
Christian Authors, Artists & Organizations: Hardbacks, Paperbacks,
eBooks, Audiobooks, Music & Film

To the Land of the Lost: Saving My Child from the Grip of Asperger's
Copyright © 2013 by Innovo Publishing LLC
All rights reserved.

No part of this publication may be reproduced, stored in a retrieval system, or transmitted in any form or by any means electronic, mechanical, photocopying, recording, or otherwise, without the prior
written permission of the author.

Library of Congress Control Number: 2013915512
ISBN 13: 978-1-61314-049-9

Cover Art by Sophie L. Davy
Cover Design & Interior Layout: by Innovo Publishing, LLC

Printed in the United States of America
U.S. Printing History

First Edition: September 2013

A story of raising a child with Asperger's syndrome,
the many difficulties faced,
and how hope came out of hopelessness

In honor of . . .

The relentless dedication of parents and organizations worldwide who help children living with Asperger's syndrome.

Parents, caregivers, sisters, brothers, aunts, uncles, grandparents, and all those who dare to care, this book is in honor of you.

And dedicated to . . .

My amazing children. Sophie, for the love you have in your heart for your brothers; James, for your compassion and strength; and Graham, for taking me on the most amazing journey. I am honored to be your mother.

My mother, Rose. You will never know how grateful I am that you loved my children as much as I do.

My sisters, Elaine, Tonya, and Sharon; my brother, David, and brother-in-law, Paschal; Aunt Imelda, Cousin Jakki and her husband, Matthew. My story would be a completely different one without your love and hands-on support.

My best friend, Paula Ryan, and her family: Roger, Aaron, and beloved Amy. I love you all so very dearly. You are always in my heart.

Dr. Helen Leader, a warm support of strength during Graham's difficult years. You are a wonderful woman.

Marianne Checkley, who gave my son dignity and hope regarding his education.

All at Aspire Ireland (www.aspireirl.org) who were always at the other end of the phone whenever I needed you.

My beloved church family in Saoirse, Dublin, and the amazing way you all encouraged me to keep pushing forward with my book. Rachael Vincent, for the richness of your friendship; Debbie Thomas, for your lovely encouragement; and Denise Mullen, for organizing the writers' group that was such a blessing to me.

Innovo Publishing, who gave me support and encouragement.

And most importantly, to Jesus, who was my sole companion during those years of isolation and who remains the One I cling to, even in good times.

Thank you.

Table of Contents

Introduction 11

1. Just Another Normal Day: Then and Now 15
2. What Is Asperger's Syndrome and What Does It Look Like? 21
3. Do All Babies Cry So Much? 25
4. Early Manifestations 29
5. Something's Not Quite Right with My Child! 31
6. My Son is Formally Assessed 37
7. The Psychologist's Report Lived Out Daily 55
8. Welcome to the World of Education and In-Patient Mental Health Units 61
9. Alternative Education 75
10. My Son Turns Eighteen 83
11. Faith Rising 85

Demographics 91
Asperger's Syndrome 93
A Note to Parents 97
Resources 99

Introduction

This is a story of a child with Asperger's syndrome, a child whose medication had little impact and for whom mainstream education ceased. The story chronicles the medical journey parents often endure while searching for a diagnosis. It's an honest view into the behavioral problems that arise at the onset of puberty when meltdowns begin. It is a candid account from the heart of a mother about the many aspects of home life that are affected by raising a child with Asperger's. It is the story of how hope was realized through faith, alternative education, and family support. Most importantly, it is the story of my son's life and the courage he had to deal with his differences.

Anyone raising a child with Asperger's syndrome can relate to the title of this book. "The land of the lost" is an accurate description of a place where freedom lacks, social networks are unreachable, and darkness shrouds one's entire day. There are so many decisions a parent has to make concerning a child with Asperger's syndrome, and incorrect choices can truly result in sending these children, who are already living on the fringes of society, to "the land of the lost."

As the mom of a child with Asperger's syndrome, I have not always had the luxury of sitting back and thinking about and planning out changes or choices. On many occasions, my choices were merely reactive responses to challenging situations. In retrospect, those decisions were the most difficult. If the "choice" turned out to be a successful one, I would feel that I should always trust my instincts, but if the choice I made turned out to be a bad one, or had the potential to be, I would begin a cycle of worry, fear, and doubt about my ability to be the kind of mother my son needed. Signs of progress seemed painstakingly slow until I realized that a good amount of positive change had come about much like the slow, constant dripping of a tap. Years of pouring in, letting go, pushing forward, stepping back, and often just scratching my head in total confusion as to what route to take next had suddenly brought dividends. And like an enormous, complicated jigsaw puzzle, my son's life finally began to come together and take shape.

It's not easy to be the sole custodian of a child's life— monitoring and managing his experiences, protecting him, nurturing him, placing him on the right educational pathway that will shape his career. This stewardship job becomes a million times more agonizing, frustrating, and difficult with a child for whom the normal systems are ineffective. During my son's childhood, I was his educational sourcing secretary, his home tutor, the one who made decisions regarding medication, and who wrestled with the challenges of his very limited diet. I spent endless days experimenting to find foods and nutrients that worked for him and that he would actually eat. I was his bodyguard and his shadow, following him from room to room when he was having a meltdown to make sure he did not accidently hurt himself. I was the liaison between him and his medical professionals, the educational system, school principals, special needs assistants, and often angry people with whom he came into contact.

For twelve long, difficult years I took my child by the hand and traveled a road where isolation and desperation were always nipping at our heels. Momentarily encouraged by a door of opportunity on the horizon, I often found it remained hard shut no matter how much I pushed against it. How desperately we longed for a place where the door would be opened and we would be found.

I often felt that I was trying to create a life for Graham, molding both him and the systems that exist in our society for raising and educating our children. It was a daunting task at best. And for all practical purposes, it was an all-consuming, unpaid "career".

I felt the life and future of my son rested almost solely upon my shoulders—that if I made an incorrect choice or decision on his behalf, I would carry the weight of having closed a door of opportunity for him to be educated, to grow with his peers, to develop, and to cope with his differences. What if I closed off too many doors of opportunity for a future outside the solitude of his bedroom? He would be a man in his 30s, alone, without peers, without an education, without a career . . . lost. In the years that I was consumed with the difficulties Graham presented and the decisions I had to make for him, I lived in constant fear of sending my child into "the land of the lost" where he might remain forever.

Chapter 1

Just Another Normal Day: Then and Now

A warm smile spreads across my face whenever I remember my young child giving a name to Asperger's syndrome. She was so small and couldn't quite curl her tongue around the words. She would pipe up, "Whatever he has, he is just Graham, and he has hamburger." She was so perceptive, even then. He was, to us, just Graham, and yes, he had "hamburger."

Little is understood about Asperger's syndrome amongst the general population. I have learned over the years to say, "He is on the autism spectrum," "He has high-functioning autism," or even, "He is highly autistic under stress and pressure." It made my life easier sometimes. I am not even sure of the precise moment when Graham grasped that he has AS. It would not be until the day of his eighteenth birthday that I would hear him eloquently describe his condition to another teenager. But during those early years of his childhood, it was incredibly difficult to explain to my son why he had to have brain scans, visit doctors and counselors, and talk with psychologists. Essentially, he knew nothing other than being who he was. I can only liken it to when people, upon hearing that I have a twin, ask, "What's it like being a twin?" to which I reply, "What's it like not?" To tell someone that he has a condition that makes him behave, think, or process emotions differently is difficult enough when the person can sit, listen, and comprehend what is being said. But with Graham, it was almost impossible to have an actual two-sided conversation, especially if it was not related to his latest hobby or obsession. It was years before he understood what Asperger's syndrome even is. I would just tell him that it made him highly intelligent, but he would need some help managing his emotions and expressing his feelings.

People would look at this very handsome young boy with chocolate brown eyes and a lovely voice and see how much he loved to chat away with adults and think that there was "not too much wrong with that child." Only those privileged enough to be with my son full time saw the many layers and facets of how the syndrome impaired and delayed his development.

A normal day then

On this particular morning, I was taking Graham with me as I delivered his little sister and brother to school. His siblings were very sweet, obedient children who never required much from me in the way of discipline; they were just so easy to manage. However, on this particular morning, Graham did not want to be taken into the school. Already I had battled and fought verbally with him for over two hours, and now, after all the stress of trying to find a parking place near the school, I had the impossible task of trying to get him out of the car so I could walk the other two children into their school. I needed to make the drop-off as quick as possible so I wouldn't get a parking violation. I had two young children who did not walk quickly and Graham, who I could not leave alone in the car. Graham began chanting, "I wanna go home, I wanna go home." It was almost impossible to reason with him once this began. As I quickened the pace, I attempted to treat him as I would any child, explaining that we were dropping off the others at their school and then I would drive him to his. I explained that it was a school day, he was up and dressed, not sick, and he needed to go, but I just could not penetrate the shroud that covered my son's ability to understand or reason. He repeated his sentence over and over again: "I wanna go home . . . I wanna go home . . . I wanna go home."

When we finally made our way into the schoolyard and almost had the younger ones delivered, Graham decided he had had enough. Here came a meltdown in full force. There in the middle of the schoolyard, with the trickling of late pupils and busy moms rushing to their next duty, he kicked me over and over again in the shins repeating, "I wanna go home, I wanna go home." It was an incredibly isolating experience, and it dawned on me how numb I had become to what people thought of me. I was used to the disapproving glances and raised eyebrows that expressed others' judgment: "What a terrible, spoiled, and bold child. I wonder what type of dysfunctional household he comes from?" But there was no invitation to help. To all in that schoolyard, Graham outwardly showed no visible sign that he was impaired by a disability. As far as they could tell, he was just a child who probably had parents who did not care enough about him to discipline him, and now he was acting like a spoiled brat, throwing tantrums. How I longed for my other two children to come back out from their classrooms and allow those parents to see how sweet, loving, and wonderfully behaved they were. That would affirm that I was a good parent.

I turned away from Graham and walked quickly away, knowing he would follow me to the car. How I wished people knew that my son was struggling with a disability that overwhelmed him sometimes. How I wished they knew him as I did; how I wished they knew me. But I could see how fearful they were. And who could blame them for not wanting to interfere? They had no idea what or why this child was as he was, nor could they have. I probably would have done the same thing—remained an onlooker.

On that day, I had one goal—to get Graham into his school. Somehow I managed to succeed despite his onslaught of angry words and lashing out, only to return home and find a message on the phone saying, "Come and pick up your son now, please." It was a message I would hear many times in the years that followed.

It was just a normal day.

A normal day now

Graham was up at 5:00 a.m., had just come downstairs slightly damp from a shower, and was offering to accompany me to a local shop for breakfast, to which I gladly obliged.

As we walked around inside the shop we had frequented for the past thirteen years, Graham asked about which pastry his sister would like and whether or not I could manage at the hot chocolate machine. As he saw a gush of hot milk pump into the oversized paper cup, he laughed at me and said, "Mom, I think you may have the wrong size cup for that hot chocolate." He was right.

A store clerk stepped from around the corner of the deli, spotted this tall young man standing beside me, and greeted him. "Hi, Graham. Wow, you're a young man now! Look at how tall you are." She recalled Graham racing to the counter and her asking him which lollipop he wanted. She marveled at how he had grown.

Graham seemed to have disappeared from these kinds of outings many years ago, when he had retreated to the safety of his home. The reaction from the store clerk was like one who sees a butterfly suddenly emerge from its cocoon. It's how many people react when they see me with my son today.

As my tall, handsome son took my heavy grocery bag, he looked every bit like a courteous, well-adjusted young man who had been taught all of his life to be a gentleman. It was just another normal day.

Parents of children with Asperger's syndrome, there is hope. It's hard to put into words all that we overcame to get to this place, but we did it, and you can do it, too.

Chapter 2

What Is Asperger's Syndrome and What Does It Look Like?

Asperger's syndrome is clinically described as impairment in social interaction. There is failure to develop peer-level friendships. This impairment includes problems understanding nonverbal communication, facial expression, and body language. Since interpreting these cues is impossible for them, people perceive them as rude, stubborn, arrogant, self-absorbed, or unintelligent. Unless they are discussing their current obsessive hobby (for Graham, this was model airplanes), conversation does not exist or is totally one-sided. This can drive people crazy and make them want to just get away. It's difficult for a parent to watch. Because I wanted to protect him from feeling confused or rejected, I became Graham's social conversation policewoman. I would stand by, listening closely, and would wind up the conversation any time I felt the other person had had enough.

Graham lived in a typical home where any child who had hurt or upset another would likely hear, "Now, how would you feel if someone did that to you?" Normally, a child would give that some thought, but Graham never did. I vividly recall the day I came to understand the lack of empathy associated with AS. I was sitting down to dinner with Graham and my other two children, James and Sophie, who were, at the time, very small. We had bought a puppy for Graham, as he was obsessed with dogs, and we felt it would be great for Graham's development to own his own dog. As we sat eating dinner, the little Jack Russell suddenly bit me hard on the ankle. I jumped out of my chair and let out a mighty screech. There was a trickle of blood running down onto my foot. James and Sophie jumped up and ran to me asking, "Mommy, Mommy, are you okay?" Graham just sat there, still, and continued to eat as if nothing had happened. Graham did eventually learn to empathize, but it would take until early adulthood.

Asperger's syndrome is an autism spectrum disorder that causes children to experience overwhelming emotions that they just cannot control. "Meltdowns" are the most difficult part of daily living. Meltdowns can manifest themselves in many ways. The child may physically fall to the floor as if he's writhing in pain. He may cry or yell with such intensity that it's hard for him to breathe. He may throw objects, hit, and kick.

With my son, meltdowns took on the worst form—rage attacks. It was never easy to pinpoint the source of his meltdown since, with Graham, there was always delayed reaction, whether it was to an environmental over-stimulation (lights, smells, sounds), an encounter with someone who had upset him, or just hormones washing over him that agitated his mind. Graham never discussed his emotions; he simply lacked the ability to process them correctly and discuss them. He would absorb all the negativity, stress, and difficulties he was experiencing until it reached the point of eruption, and oftentimes over a simple or senseless issue. I spent years trying to devise a coping strategy to help Graham, and all of us, to live with these rage eruptions. It was like living in a war zone. Whenever I sensed that a meltdown was about to occur, I would phone my sister, who knew to come and collect my two little ones and take them to the safety of her house until Graham's outburst had ended. Hours later, when everything was back to normal, I would begin cleaning up the mess he had created and wonder how on earth he would ever be able to live with this condition.

If you are a parent whose child has meltdowns, know that you are not alone. It does end and life does stabilize . . . eventually. If your child does not suffer with meltdowns, realize how blessed you are and be thankful for one less challenge you have to deal with.

It was often in the late hours of the evening when I would cry pitifully, begging God for help. I would fall into bed exhausted and covered in bruises from having interceded or been caught in the crossfire of my son's outbursts. With red, swollen eyes from the tears of the night before and hurting knees, another day would begin—and with it, another potential meltdown. I would smack a huge smile on my face, have my morning coffee, get my little ones up for their school day, and kiss them and cuddle them as if all was right with the world. I had to. And when Graham got up, I would greet him with a smile and say, "Good morning, Son, how are you, my love?" This was the best way to give him dignity and unconditional love, to boost his self-esteem. I learned that in the same way a mother cleans up after a child who has been sick, without holding him accountable or reminding him of the terrible mess he made, that is how meltdowns should be handled.

I would become an expert in living and dealing with Asperger's syndrome, but early on, I hadn't a clue what I was doing. Oh, how I longed for a "super nanny" who was specially trained in managing the challenges of Asperger's syndrome. I could have saved myself from the wounds of guilt over how I handled my son with such lack of understanding. Today, when I see a child with Asperger's syndrome, I want to take his parents in my arms and tell them all the things I learned the hard way and give them hope.

Chapter 3

Do All Babies Cry So Much?

I was working in financial services and had fallen in love with a consultant from London who was drafted to help us set up a new operations hub in the financial sector. I still can remember thinking to myself, *I've never believed in love at first sight, but this must be what it feels like.* Within months, I became pregnant. Soon after that, the company sent my baby's father back to London. All contact ceased between us. Pregnant, single, but with a good income to raise my child alone, I moved out of my family home and into a rental with a close friend of mine.

With the birth of Graham came my first experience in motherhood. I remember the first time I saw his little face as I lay on the labor and delivery bed in the hospital. Having given one mighty push, shaken and exhausted, I lifted my head, and as I peered down at him, his black eyes stared back at mine and penetrated my heart. It *was* love at first sight—a moment I would never forget.

Graham began to cry within hours of my taking him home. I nursed him constantly, and I was exhausted. He had to be rocked to sleep, and my arms ached so much. One night he lost his breath and turned blue, so I rushed him to the hospital. There he was attached to heart monitors, and whenever I would enter the room and he would hear me, his little heart would beat faster, responding to my voice. It was in moments like that when I believed I was born to be a mother.

I returned home, my son being given the all-clear as a normal, healthy child. But Graham's crying and screaming continued. I remember thinking, *How does any woman actually have another child?* Since I was a first-time mother, I had no idea that this crying fell far outside the normal behavior of an infant. After about twelve hours of non-stop howling and squirming, I drove frantically to the hospital and begged them to tell me what was wrong with my child. My brother-in-law and twin sister were with me as we watched the doctors check my baby boy. We left with a diagnosis of colic. I knew there was something more; I just did not know then that his world was so very different than mine—that lights hurt his eyes, sounds overwhelmed him, smells were too strong for him, and clothes and blankets were irritating against his delicate skin.

Had I known then what was to come concerning this child, would I even have believed it? Could I have imagined this little black-eyed baby someday intentionally and repeatedly smashing his head against walls? How would I have felt knowing I would spend years physically restraining this child so he would not harm himself or others? Would I have believed that he would come to routinely destroy everything he could possibly spill, break, or throw in our house and then curl up in a fetal position and rock himself back into calm? What would I have thought of the woman who would drive with this child and her other two, as he kicks, bites, and squeals at the top of his voice? How would I have felt seeing how ill fitted he would be in school system and how I would have to literally carry him into the school until finally withdrawing him in the third grade? What if I had known I would have to endure years of doctors diagnosing and analyzing every detail of our lives and Graham's behavior? Of course, I knew none of that at the time. I only remember embracing my precious infant son and envisioning how he would grow to be a happy child with lots of friends. He would be well adjusted at school, play football, and just be a regular kid.

In those early months as a mom, I never dreamed this child would take me on such an incredible journey—a long, difficult journey that neither of us expected to take, one with little preparation and one that would span many years—but we would travel it together, hand in hand, my son and me.

Chapter 4

Early Manifestations

My mother laughs now as she remembers a walk around our neighborhood with her only grandson, then two years old. It would take hours as he stopped at every single drain. His fascination with the drains would be replaced with church bells. He wanted to be taken to see them, over and over again.

During those early years, his fixations and repetitive behaviors were continuous—drains, bells, fire engines, construction trucks, lining up his toys in a row. I found this behavior difficult to deal with. After the birth of my second child, there was little room in my busy schedule to constantly cater to his fixations. He could not "leave" a fixation until he was "done." My patience grew thin when I had to run to the grocery store or my new daughter needed to get home for her feeding.

When I was utterly drained and exhausted as a young mom was when Graham's tantrums began to emerge. Once, when he was three years old, I needed to run an unexpected errand and so did not take the usual route home. He became so distressed, I gave up and turned the car around. I concluded at the time that I guess we had spoiled him.

I really didn't enjoy many of his early days. He was draining. I remember the guilt of feeling relieved when he was tucked into bed asleep or when someone else was taking him out for a walk. He was so difficult. And his sleeping pattern, even back then, was every parent's nightmare. He never seemed to be able to sleep. This was the hardest part of being with Graham exhaustion and sleep deprivation. This child just did not seem to be able to go to sleep. This would last for a decade of his life. I spent many years sitting on the stairs of his bedroom, crying my eyes out, dreading another night of putting him to bed while my other two children slept soundly in their beds. Where did I go wrong with Graham? What else do parents do but automatically blame themselves?

Chapter 5

Something's Not Quite Right with My Child!

Kindergarten

By now I was married to Graham's dad, and two more children had been added to our growing family—Sophie in 1996 followed by James in 1998. Because my husband was frequently away on business trips, my mother would make the long trip from her house to mine just to let me have a nap every day. Graham's inability to get to sleep left me worn out physically. I held onto the hope that what many mothers had said about their children's tantrums and sleeping problems being resolved once they started school would be the case with Graham. I had hoped school would be a place where he could channel his energy and intelligence and come home full and satisfied. I truly believed that Graham's difficulties at home stemmed from the lack of an outlet for his above-average intelligence and unquenchable thirst for knowledge.

During that first week of kindergarten, Graham tried hard to settle in. When two weeks had passed without incident, I believed that perhaps his behavioral problems had come to an end, but it wasn't long before problems began to surface. Recently Graham recounted vivid memories from that first year of school. He remembers being in the classroom and wanting to learn more about computers. The teacher, probably exasperated by his rapid fire of questions, had her work cut out for her! I can imagine him becoming quite annoyed when she would not (or could not) satisfy his inquiring mind and tried to grind his questioning to a halt. Deciding he was "too loud," she removed Graham from the classroom and placed him in the hallway. He wound up running out of the school. His teacher had no idea why a boy his age would not be afraid to go against what a teacher had told him to do—to stand in the hallway—in order to leave the school building and head outside alone. Few five-year-old children would have done this. It was baffling to all of us. He was such an incredibly intelligent child, yet he did not seem to grasp the concept of danger. This child who had so much fear of little things—fear of clowns, fear of taking journeys that were not planned and explained in advance—showed no fear of doing something that was actually quite dangerous.

At the middle of the school year, I sat down to talk with Graham's teacher. Although she described him as a happy, well liked, bubbly young child, who chatted to everyone and was academically showing signs of being way above his peers, she also noted that he seemed to be struggling with issues he could not comprehend or cope with. There was something about Graham that was not like the other children, but she could not identify what it was. Neither of us could understand why he had appeared to have settled into school, only to suddenly *not* settle into school. I shrugged it off thinking it would all work out. I was wrong.

Since my husband traveled abroad for his work and was home only every other weekend, I was virtually a single parent. I bought a house for the children and me closer to my family, and my husband and I officially separated the following year.

Senior Infants[1]

Graham began attending a new school. We had a new house, I was near my family, and I had three young, bright, happy children to look after. I thought life would sail along nicely for me and my little brood. On his first day of school, I remember running from the classroom where I had dropped Graham off and racing to the window to catch a glimpse of him in class. The principal saw me and disapproved. Years later, he would tell me that he used that story in conferences to tell other parents what *not* to do when dropping a child off on their first day.

In our wonderful world of child-friendly education where educators place the well-being of the child first and academics second, Graham's quirky ways were catered to, without any of us knowing he had Asperger's syndrome. We just chalked it up to his tender age and determined he simply needed security and comfort. Every day, he would go into school wearing a firefighter's costume, complete with yellow helmet. The school would accommodate him. Graham was liked by his classmates. He was a leader in the playground, directing and taking the lead in all the make-believe games he invented. These games normally revolved around his limited interests, and he fit well into this group of five year olds. But underneath lay a need for him to have order and control over all the games he invented. Everyone had his or her place and purpose. I often wondered how he actually enjoyed the make-believe games. He spent so much time watching over people, ensuring they were compliant in doing the exact task he had told them to do. I found it endearing that he had such good leadership qualities at that time. It never crossed my mind that he could not bend outside of these controls, this need inside of him. He was five. No one noticed. How could we have?

---

[1] In Ireland, "senior infants" is a school year between kindergarten and the first grade.

Inklings of differences begin to form in my mind

Bearing Sophie and James was the catalyst that gave me the first inkling that something was not quite right with my eldest son. He was an extremely intelligent child, reading beyond his age level at a very young age. My husband and I thought that we had just poured so much time into him that we had somehow probably increased Graham's intelligence. My husband had come from an academic background where his father had attended both Harvard and Oxford, so there was a bit of pride about Graham's budding higher-than-average IQ.

I viewed Graham differently than my husband. I found him to be exhausting and difficult. He was six years old and a stunningly beautiful child with silky brown hair, washed and groomed, and sallow skin with dark, chocolate brown eyes. But as beautiful a child as he was, Graham's behavior had developed slowly into every parent's worst nightmare.

Although I had reunited with Graham's dad, our marriage, which was shaky even before, was now crumbling. Our views were so vastly different. He was certain that discipline was the issue. I felt with my heart and believed that something in Graham was developing differently—very, very differently.

Seven years of Graham's life passed, and with each year he was becoming increasingly difficult to manage. I wish I could say his problems were just behavioral, but there were vast developmental and social differences from his peers in school, and his obsessive interests and problems with sleep did not seem to pass as he grew. I was very concerned with his lack of concentration, which seemed to cause his eyes to glaze over, and he would appear to go off to "some other place" momentarily. My husband noticed this too and relayed it to a neurologist.

The doctor completed initial tests in her office as we sat there in her private care consultation room. Graham appeared nervous, and when he was nervous, he would revert to behaving like a toddler. He acted silly. He swung his arms and paced the room, going from one object to another asking questions about each of the objects in a monotonous tone. At one point, Graham was lying down on the floor, rolling from side to side. I remember being embarrassed, as I did not feel we were in a child-friendly consultation. Graham was ignored as we concentrated on all the information we could give the doctor about our son's strange behaviors.

This doctor never told me what she believed was causing Graham's development differences; she merely referred to him to a psychologist. Our family doctor received a letter from her which read:

> *Graham did not have any abnormal neurological signs. Hyperventilation for more than 200 breaths failed to induce an absence (mild epilepsy). He presented as a boy with some features of Attention Deficit Disorder and I did not think he was classical Asperger's, although he still could have that condition. I am arranging an EEG with hyperventilation to make sure he does not have absence epilepsy, and I will let you know the results in due course.*

It would be five years before I ever saw a copy of this letter, so we never knew that the neurologist saw Graham presenting ADD and Asperger's syndrome. Although she mentioned he was having ongoing assessments regarding both, we were never aware of any of it. It was one of those invaluable pieces of information—early detection—that may have changed the course of Graham's educational and Asperger's needs.

Chapter 6

My Son Is Formally Assessed

Three years had passed since I had initially sought to understand if there was a specific cause for Graham's peculiarities and behavior. He would run wildly through the house, squealing and flapping his arms until they looked like they might dislodge from their sockets. All the while, he would be hysterically laughing. His eyes would glaze over, and he would grab anything in his pathway, even once taking a water gun and aiming it at the lights that hung down from the ceiling. I could see him heading full force with the water gun aimed at the electric lights, and I was petrified!

   Graham's outbursts of wildness were an everyday occurrence. Their frequency was exhausting. The rage outbursts that fell immediately on the tail of the wild outbursts were the worst thing I have ever experienced in my life, and my heart melts with empathy for any parent who is in the midst of these challenges. I wish I could tell you I was the perfect mother, calm and in control, but I cannot. At times like this, when I thought he or someone else was in danger, I would chase him, shouting hysterically while every other child present would scatter, start crying, or cower in a corner for fear of this tornado. But nothing would halt him. I would inadvertently leave red marks on his exposed arms where I grabbed him. Every time I raced after Graham, my voice raising in pitch as it fell on the deafened ears of my son in the height of his outburst, I hated who I had become.

Slowly, feelings of inadequacy, which would plague me for years to come, began to give rise to a wound that had cut so deeply it changed how I viewed myself. Very few people touch upon the subject of caregivers' emotional well-being and the damage it causes to one's psyche and self-esteem. It crushes it. Even books on Asperger's syndrome or people who deal with children with behavioral challenges don't really dive into the life of the caregiver. It is an issue lacking transparency.

With the original understanding of Asperger's syndrome—that the parents were to blame—I felt as if I was under an intense microscope and had to constantly defend myself against this mindset so it would not take hold of me also, as it would have lain me so low that I would have given up completely. My heart would have died if ever I had thought that I had caused my son's difficulties. I adored him and nurtured him and had cherished him from the very moment he was born. My heart was torn into so many pieces when I saw the condition he lived in, inside of himself, without seeming to have the ability to be "normal." I felt so eternally grateful that I had two other children in my life; they were an anchor of reality for me, with their normal development, normal play patterns, self-control, and gentleness. I clung to this tiny flicker of belief in myself as a good, nurturing mother. For years, in the quietness of the evening when my children were fast asleep, I would sit and just cup my hands over my face and let out sobs so deep that I often felt that if sorrow had a voice, it would certainly be that sound. Tears and my faith in God, the only One who ever heard those sobs, were my evening companions for all of those long years. And so my faith in God grew while faith in myself diminished.

Graham bubbles to a bursting point! My first cry for medical intervention

Children with Asperger's syndrome find it incredibly difficult to articulate their emotions or describe incidents. On the days he successfully managed to remain in school, as I collected him, I would strike up a conversation with him asking, "How did your day go, Son?" If he responded at all, he would use one syllable to describe it and then motion for me to get him home. I think of the joy of collecting my other two children from school. Whenever I asked them about their day, they would hold my hand and chatter excitedly until we arrived back home. I would hear of how Joe hit Rachael in the schoolyard and got into big trouble, or how they had painted a picture of spring, or glued more pieces of paper onto their class collage. This only emphasized how different Graham was in his interaction with the world and his inability to carry on a normal conversation.

I was unaware of the stress Graham was under at school. Not only was he being bullied over his repetitive games, but his motorized, repetitive fixations were also being considered bullying by other children. Also there was a serious incident in the schoolyard where children were subjected to having their trousers pulled down by some of the other students. I learned that Graham had been a victim of this schoolyard prank, though he never did voice his feelings about the matter. His only expression was a complete meltdown, which would come days or sometimes weeks later.

One day Graham took a kitchen knife out of the drawer and held it to his stomach. As I stood beside him, he said, "I will do it . . . I will stab myself." On this particular day, it was as if all his stress had bubbled to the surface and exploded. Even if Graham did not have the ability to articulate or to express his thoughts and feelings, he was not immune to emotional damage to his heart and mind. As Graham reached for the only object he could find in the kitchen drawer, he had come to breaking point. The emotionally silent world in which he lived had come to a head, and he was channeling all his negative experiences into the one emotion he could express—rage.

As he held the knife to hurt himself, I knew he was in a great deal of emotional pain. Having completed an eighteen-month basic training course in Christian counseling, I grasped at every ounce of knowledge I had stored away and replied as quickly as the words could form in my mouth. "You can, Son," I said slowly and calmly. "You can stab yourself, but you may not succeed in killing yourself. You might damage your body in a way that would mean you will have to spend the rest of your life in a wheelchair, or you may lose the ability to use your arms. Playing Legos or your using your computer would not be an option." Graham appeared to be mulling over this vivid picture I had presented of the consequences of harming himself. He quickly put the knife down. Outwardly, I may have appeared calm and composed, but inside, my heart was pounding, and there was little color left in my face. Graham's face was so sad. I knew deep down, somewhere in the recesses of his heart and mind, he was in pain. And there was not one part of me that did not ache to protect him from the emotional damage and low self-esteem brought on by the challenging behaviors associated with Asperger's syndrome.

I decided it was time to withdraw Graham from school temporarily and to seek urgent medical intervention.

The visit to my GP . . . and a meltdown. I wanted answers!

The next morning, Graham and I sat in the general practitioner's office while I told her what had happened. She agreed that he needed urgent intervention and gave me a referral letter for Graham to be assessed by a psychologist.

Graham had "sticky thought processing," where the brain gets a thought in it and simply cannot let go until it is acted upon. Whenever Graham decided he wanted something, it made little difference if it was an impossible request. Once the thought was in his head, it would drive him almost insane until the item was retrieved, found, purchased, or whatever. More often than not, I would give in; it was easier, and I knew where it would lead if I didn't.

As we left the doctor's office, Graham wanted a gumball. I had no money with me, and I explained this to Graham. "I want a gumball, . . . I want a gumball," he chanted incessantly. He had always gotten a gumball when he visited the doctor, and I was breaking routine. Finally, we were back to the car and heading home. I was feeling good that I had secured that referral letter I needed. Suddenly Graham began to kick the dashboard of the car until it broke. I was horrified. As I tried to stop him, he stretched out his arms, wildly flapping and kicking, and I got caught in the crossfire of his kicks and thrashing. I could not believe this was happening. It's strange the things one's mind recalls when memories of intense pleasure or pain are experienced. But I remember sitting in the car, looking out the window, with a child kicking, hitting, and grunting, and trying to dive and escape the onslaught. I thought, *Does anyone see what is happening? This is not normal.* Amazingly, no one seemed to notice anything, or if they did, they didn't approach the car. At last I started home, my hair in a tangled mess. I was shaken. When we got home, Graham quietly found a room, curled up into a ball, and rocked himself. I was still trembling as I made a cup of tea and reached for a cigarette. I was in shock. What was happening to us?

These outbursts would become a normal part of our day and escalate severely over the coming years. And after every meltdown, my beautiful, intelligent son would rock himself on the floor in a fetal position. How I longed to pick him up, as I did when he was little, and tell him everything would be okay, but he could not handle being touched or held. My words were the only way I could "hold" and hug my son.

Before we saw the psychologist, I was to begin collecting documentation related to Graham's daily struggles and behavior. This proved to be quite an arduous task spanning four years. The school principal was well aware of and involved in Graham's school avoidance, tantrums, and outbursts. He even came to my house one morning as a concerned fatherly figure trying to help a young, struggling mother. He found Graham, eyes glazed over and laughing hysterically, crouched under the kitchen table where he remained for the entire visit. He was unsuccessful in coaxing Graham to come to school. I think that was a turning point in his understanding that something was not right with this ten-year-old. I received the following letter from him a few days later, which was the first letter added to my documentation collection.

> *Graham has attended this primary school since junior infants.*[2] *Since starting here, he presented as a very shy and introverted boy who was slow to participate in group activities. He does not make friends easily and has only one close friend in school.*
>
> *He comes across, at times, as being quite immature emotionally, while at the same time intellectually functioning quite highly. School work is good, generally speaking. However, he misses quite a lot of school, which ultimately is going to be detrimental to his future progress. Much of this time missed is due to "tantrums" where he refuses to come into school when his mother has gone to the trouble of presenting him at school. This is getting progressively worse and seriously needs to be addressed.*
>
> *We in the school feel that Graham needs a psychological assessment as soon as possible. We are more concerned about his emotional development than his academic progress, as he appears to*

---

[2] In Ireland, "junior infants" is equivalent to kindergarten in the US.

be developing a "victim complex"—everything to him appears to be bullying whereas it usually is not. His self-esteem appears seriously low and I would be worried he might harm himself eventually.

Armed with this recommendation, we were appointed our first meeting with a psychologist. I was so relieved. I thought Graham would be treated, and life would normalize. How little I knew back then. I am glad I knew so little. My husband came with us to that first meeting; it was the only time he would attend any meeting with his son.

The first psychologist, one of many

Graham was kept amused outside while we sat in a little room with wall-to-wall children's drawings. Being a young man in his mid-twenties, the psychologist was so enthusiastic. A full history was taken of Graham. I felt stripped and slightly awkward as I recounted all of Graham's development milestones, his rapidly escalating meltdowns, and his rage and hysteria episodes. Later, as I gazed at Graham, I felt such betrayal that I wanted to weep. It was difficult to discuss the private struggles of my son in this environment and with a stranger. I wanted to tell the young psychologist all of Graham's good qualities—the lovely things he did to make me laugh and the way he could build the most complicated Lego *Star Wars* spaceship without using the instructions. He was amazing. Yet we were not there to tell of his victories—only the things we were not coping with. I had to recount the day we bought that Lego spaceship after he had hounded me for days. By the time we got to the store to purchase the toy, with his level of excitement high and the store's fluorescent lights, he became wild with excitement, and I had to carry this now very heavy ten-year-old out of the store. Once the spaceship was completed, his fixation and hounding would begin all over again.

I believe my husband thought Graham was just spoiled and that I was not a good parent, that I was fueling his behavior. I was of a very different opinion. Graham's outbursts were so much easier to deal with than the rift between my husband and me. As we sat in that little room talking with the psychologist, I knew we were holding onto the very last thread of our marriage.

Graham had many sessions with the young psychologist, who I later learned was only in training before writing his thesis. The doctor was so intrigued by Graham's presentation that he would go on to complete his thesis on Graham and Asperger's syndrome. This young doctor was the first person Graham touched because of his condition. He would inspire many others in the years to come.

When the battery of appointments had concluded, the first comprehensive report was completed. Another psychologist commented later that it was the most comprehensive report she had ever seen and that parents seldom get this type of detailed analysis. Even before it was written, I had scoured books and the Internet and had already concluded that Asperger's syndrome was present in Graham. An excerpt from the report, having taken a few months to complete through analyzing Graham and us as a family, reads as follows:

Reason for Referral:

Graham was referred to the Department of Psychology in the Health Centre by his GP. Graham was referred for school refusal, stubbornness, being withdrawn and episodes of rage. It was reported that Graham was both being bullied and bullying others at school. He has displayed highly aggressive behavior at home, physically lashing out. He also threatened to harm himself with a kitchen knife in his hand. A tentative early diagnosis of epilepsy was mentioned and the GP noted he was being referred to a pediatrician to establish if this is present or not. His mother mentioned that Graham had exhibited difficulty in learning math, and given Graham's behavioral difficulties in school and intellectual assessment to check for specific learning disabilities was deemed appropriate.

Presentation of Child:

Graham presented as playful, friendly, sociable, and energetic. He was curious about the room he found himself in, commenting on art work on the wall, noting the types of painting instruments used to create the pictures. He said that he was interested in doing painting or modeling clay or drawing and we agreed to do this next time on his appointment visit to the clinic.

Sleep Pattern:

Graham would stay up late and complained of not being tired at bedtime. . . . He reported having difficulty seeing depth perception and he says he "sees things sometimes in black and white." He is being referred currently to an eye surgeon.

External Stimuli:

I discussed with the parents and they explained that Graham has always disliked loud noises. He also dislikes strong smells. His mother reports that he "hates the smell of people." Graham will often block his ears to loud sounds and becomes upset when he is in a place (e.g. large shop) with high visual stimulation.

Anger Outbursts:

Graham has a history of angry outbursts, sometimes culminating in violent attacks of rage on his mother. Graham's mother has difficulty discerning what triggers these outbursts, but does notice that when it is about to happen his mood and tone of voice change. These outbursts are coupled with intense "irrational fears" that result in Graham cowering in a corner or hiding underneath tables or beds.

Graham is reported as often being kind and very caring, but will interrupt conversations. Graham often bullies his little sister, in particular a target of his outbursts, and has difficulties with relationships. He will incite bullying behavior in other children by behaving agitating or aggressively towards them. . . . Graham exhibits problems in observing social cues e.g. turn taking in conversation, persistence in talking when other desists with interaction.

Performance Abilities:

The performance score provides an indication of an individual's non-verbal reasoning, spatial skills, attentiveness to detail and visual motor integration. Graham's non-verbal reasoning skills are in the high average range and better than 84% of his peers. Graham scored highest in the picture arrangement. . . .This would suggest strengths in visual perception and complete meaningful stimuli, visual organization, and anticipation of consequences, temporal sequencing and time concepts. . . . Graham scored low on coding; however, this difference is not significant. Test behavior of attention to detail and perfectionism may account for this lower score. This subtest represents a measure of executive functioning that is often a deficit in Asperger's children.

Processing Speed Abilities:

The PSI provides a measure of an individual's ability to process simple or routine visual information quickly and efficiently and to quickly perform tasks based on that information. Graham's skill in processing visual material without making errors is comparable to that of his peers. His performance on the PSI was better than 34% of his age cohorts. This was Graham's lowest index score. A relative weakness in processing speed may make the task of comprehending novel information more time consuming and difficult for Graham.

Freedom from Distractibility Index:

The FDI measures ability to remain free from distraction. Graham's score on this is comparable to that of his peers. This suggests Graham can maintain concentration and appears to have low levels of distractibility.

Summary:
Graham's general cognitive ability is in the high average range of intellectual functioning.

His overall thinking and reasoning abilities exceed those of approximately 84% of peers his age. This would suggest that Graham has considerable abilities on which to rely in a learning environment. The performance score provides an indication of an individual's non-verbal reasoning, spatial skills, and attentiveness to detail.

Children with Asperger's syndrome are often of high intelligence. However, the profiles are often uneven, as is with Graham. His unique profile is indicative of particular areas of strengths and weaknesses that are likely to manifest in unique learning needs. Graham's tendency to obsess about particular objects or subjects may interrupt his learning; however, attempts should be made to integrate these interests into his learning. For example using "Star Wars" figures in comprehension stories to generate motivation. Graham exhibits high general knowledge for factual information. In the interests of maintaining motivation, this ability should be recognized and praised when appropriate. Graham's reported difficulty in engaging in social groups suggest a need for some one on one work time, as well as some social interaction.

Screening Used for the Detection of the Presence of Asperger's Syndrome:
Bender Gestalt Screening for Neurological Dysfunction
Connors Parent Behavior Rating Scale
Screening Questionnaire for Asperger's Syndrome
Australian Scale for Asperger's Syndrome

Summary:

Graham appears to be exhibiting many of the characteristics of Asperger's syndrome. He is also exhibiting challenging behaviors, which are likely strongly associated with the presence of Asperger's syndrome and not necessarily indicative of a separate disorder. Graham does not appear to exhibit perceptual or neurological difficulties.

End of Report.

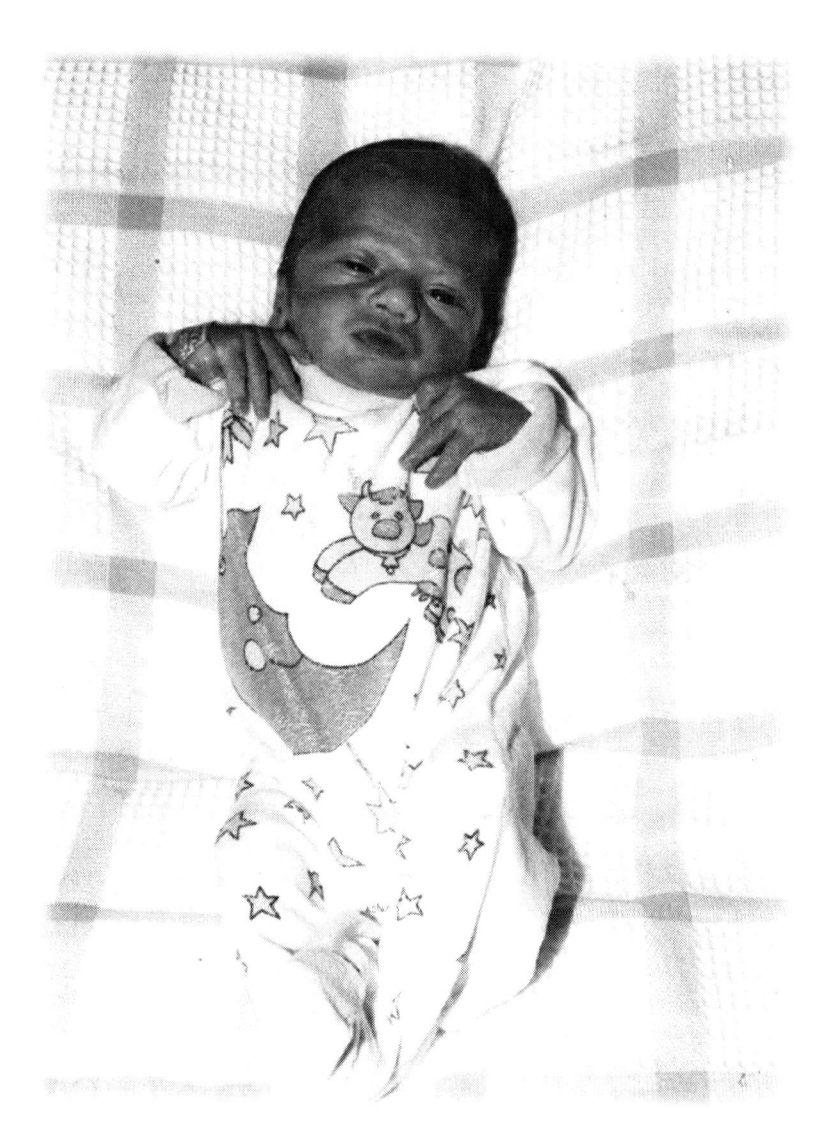

My "black-eyed boy" (Graham, two days old)

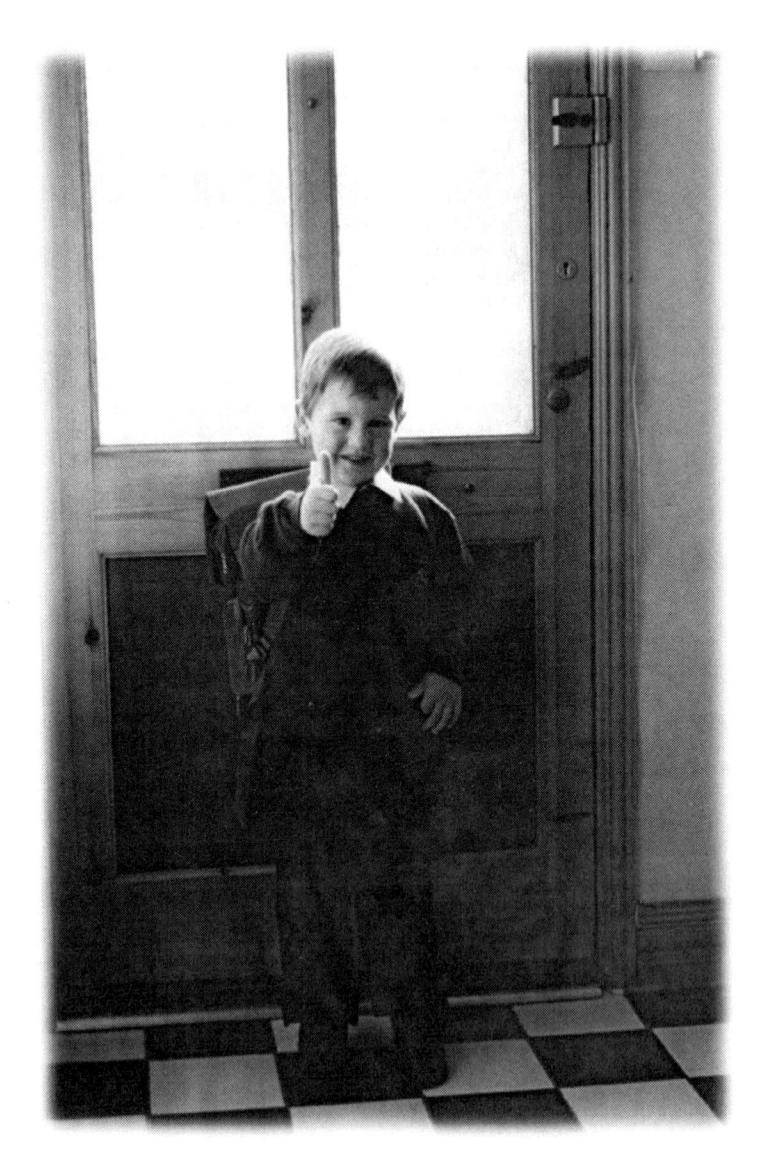

First day of elementary school!

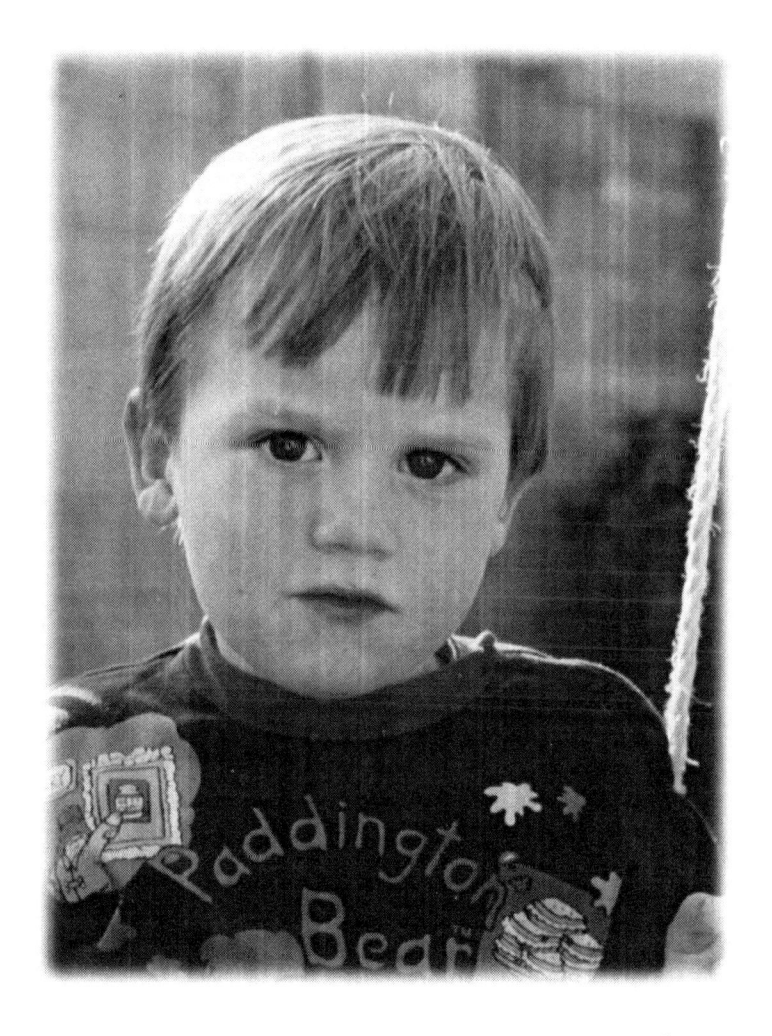

Those chocolate brown eyes . . . (two years old)

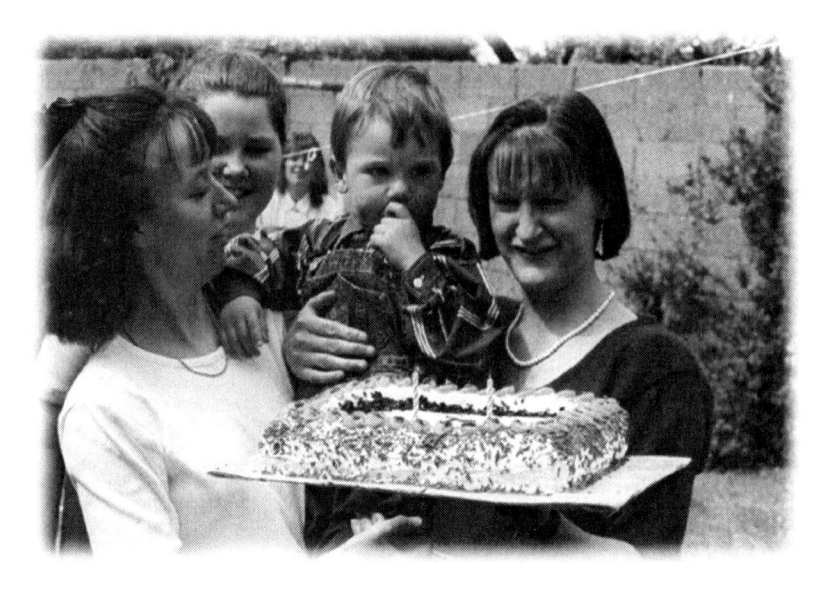

Overwhelmed by the noise. Graham's second birthday party
(with my twin sister, Tonya)

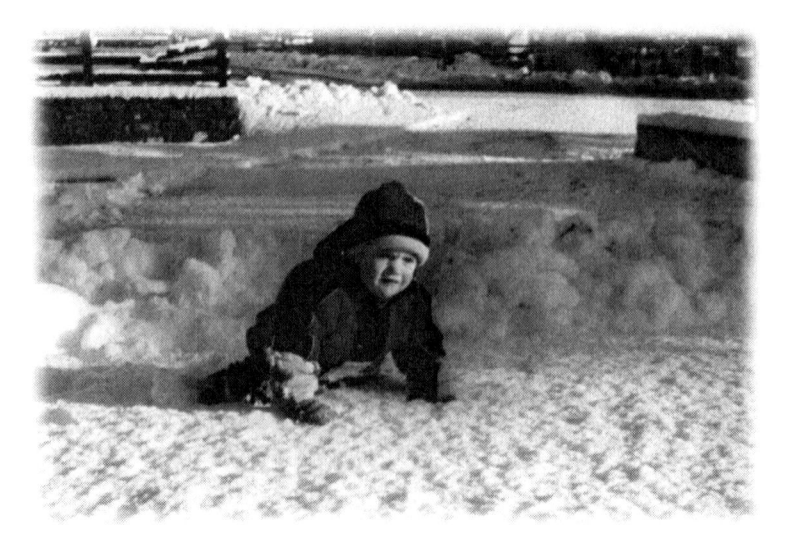

Graham hating snow!

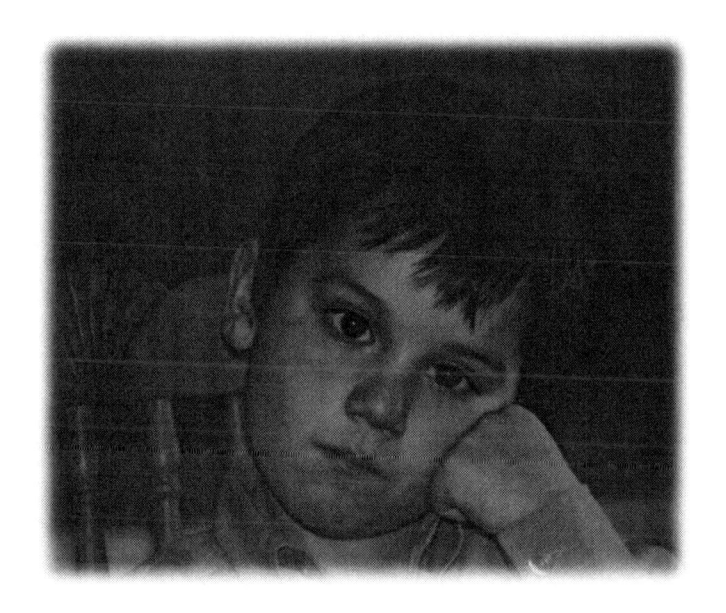

Graham looking distant

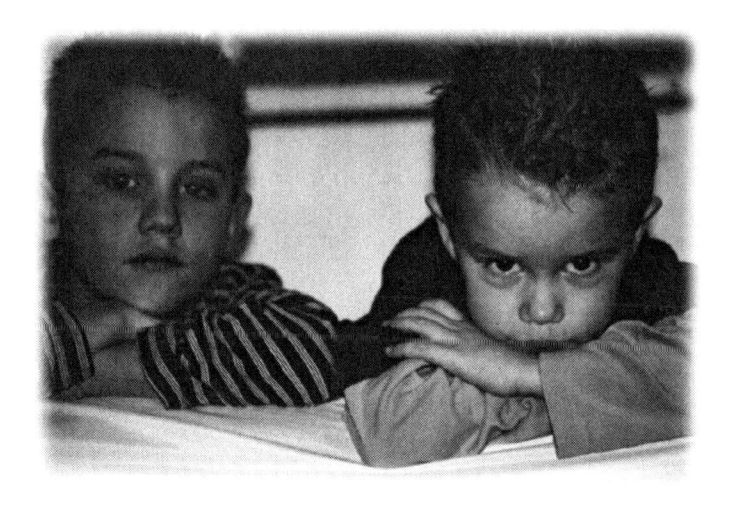

That "glazed-eye look" that always seemed to be in Graham's beautiful eyes

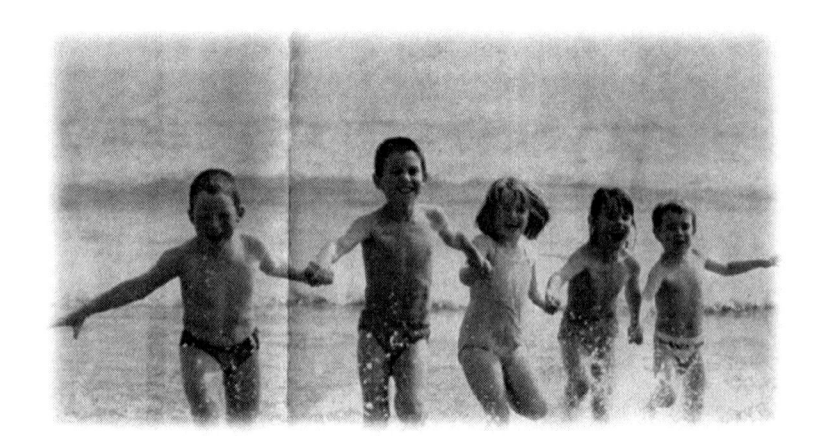

Graham, Aaron, Amy, Sophie, and James.
At the height of his "meltdowns," life went on.

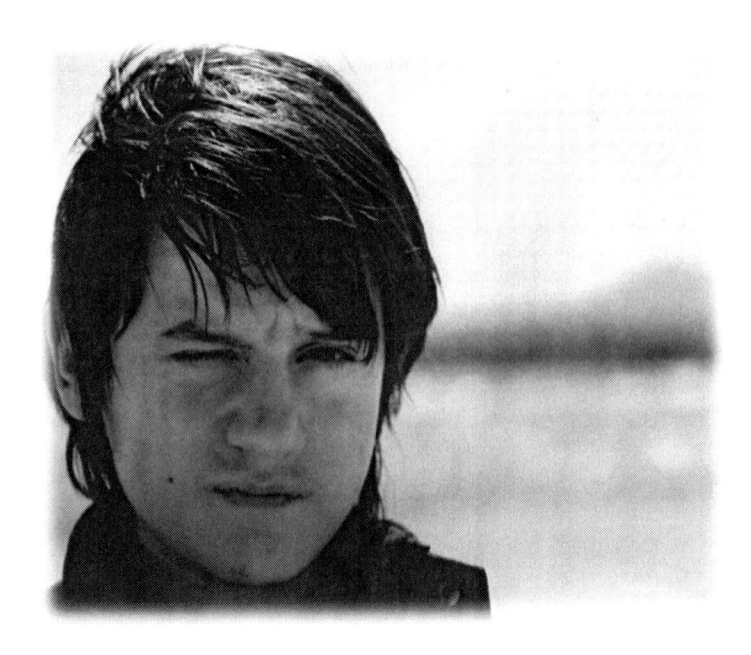

My precious Graham, age 15

Chapter 7

The Psychologist's Report Lived Out Daily

Although I was thrilled when Graham was at school, sometimes, in all truth, I was relieved when the school holidays came around because I got a break from the stress of trying to get Graham into school and remain there. I was exhausted, frustrated, and it was all anyone ever seemed to ask me—did Graham go to school? In hindsight, I placed too much pressure on Graham during those years because of the pressure I was under. But if I didn't even try to get him into school, who would? By this time, my husband and I had been separated for some time, and we would eventually legally divorce a few years later.

Graham was difficult at home. He had to be watched almost 100 percent of the time. I always felt edgy and decided I most certainly had some form of Post-Traumatic Stress Disorder. I sought help for Sophie and James to voice their feelings about the unpredictable mood swings and meltdowns they had to live with. It was a daily occurrence for me to tell them, "Go to your rooms and lock yourselves in." They would retreat to safety until I called them again when Graham's meltdown was over. I would then begin the task of calming him and quietly cleaning up the mess that had been created.

As Graham grew in age and strength, cumulative unresolved stressors would trigger hysteria and repetitive, motorized behavior. I only had to look at my son's arms flapping and his glazed eyes to know he was in a place of great distress, and his emotions were about to burst wide open. The tension of my everyday life was at times unbearable. I could not recall what it was like to live without feeling on edge.

I dreaded sunny days. I would awake in the morning, and the first thing I would do is check the weather. If it was raining, I was relieved; it meant Graham would not want to go outside and play—a problem I would not have to deal with. Parents of children with learning or social challenges can empathize with this relief. I was acutely aware that while professionals and close friends and family were supportive, some people were not. Occasionally neighbors would come storming over, simply irate with my son's behavior. I was not well equipped to deal with angry neighbors. Once Graham had taken something from another child. He had seen an object and decided it was his, the one he had lost. There was no reasoning with Graham once he got something into his head; it just seemed to make him more adamant that he was right and everyone else was wrong. Graham held the object, a toy gun, in the hallway while this neighbor screamed at me. I tried to calm the situation, but all the while, I wanted to scream at Graham to give back whatever he had taken, regardless of whether it was his or not. Every day brought so many calamities that I just wanted to lock the world out. I could endure the long hours of Graham's meltdowns on my own ground, safely behind the confines of our home, but when it spilled over to other people, especially hot-tempered adults, I just could not cope with that. It cut me deeply to hear such anger and frustration directed at my son. This was my child whom I had borne and dearly loved. I wanted to tell her that he was doing his best to overcome the challenges of living with AS, but it was not the time.

Graham's perception and understanding were very slanted. Even if adults saw what had happened in a situation, Graham would recount a very different story. He never changed the event details; he just perceived them differently. He always felt he was in the right, and he would constantly defend his position. He tended to only see his side of an argument, could not place himself into another person's shoes, and did not know how to read nonverbal language. On one particular occasion, Graham was on his friend's case constantly. To everyone it was clear that Graham was deliberately provoking the boy, and when he could take it no longer, he physically attacked Graham. That's when Graham started his rant: "I have done nothing!" Graham seemed to truly believe this too. He believed he had done nothing—that the boy was annoying him—and he would look puzzled as to why he would want to hit him.

Sometimes Graham would take an instant, unexplainable disliking to someone, such as the little girl across the street, who enjoyed coming over to play with Sophie. This is common with children who have Asperger's syndrome; they can just dislike someone, and that's that. Often I ended up shouting at Graham for pushing the girl simply "because I don't like her!" There would be no provocation; Graham would just act out. He loved to terrorize children with his remote-controlled car. Even if others protested for him to stop steering it into the back of their legs, he continued.

Graham also had a way of verbally pounding a person until he reached his breaking point. This was a huge problem; he constantly irritated other people by deliberately winding them up. When people thought he was being mean, he thought he was being funny. As is the case with most children with AS, Graham had a wacky sense of humor. Sometimes I watched him use it as a defense mechanism for situations he could not cope with or process. He had feelings, and they could be hurt; he just displayed them differently.

The daily life of Asperger's syndrome was taking its toll on me

It's not easy to teach things to a child with Asperger's syndrome that his peers seem to just know. Even though it was my job to chastise him for his behavior, I knew that Graham lacked understanding and needed a constant resource at his side to prompt him concerning what was or was not acceptable. I deeply empathized with him. I was fully aware of his capabilities and limitations. For years, I would pull up a chair to our large living room window and sit there ready to run outside whenever intervention was needed. On many occasions I would hustle Graham inside and take the verbal abuse myself. I couldn't defend my son, nor was there any point in explaining why he was the way he was. Angry people have little or no empathy.

Graham's favorite way of describing anyone who said something to upset him was, "They're mean!" and he would dislike them intensely from that time forward. For that reason, I tried to shield Graham from any individual who I felt would not make allowances for his behavior.

The corrosive effect of Asperger's syndrome takes years to be mended and restored. Seven years after Graham's diagnosis, I did not even recognize the person I had become. I lived on the edge of fear, not knowing what each day would bring—a meltdown? an angry, screaming neighbor? a sobbing child whom Graham had agitated? more bruises from the physical wrestling? Only one thing was certain: I always knew that there would be sobbing in the evening; it's when my mind would travel to far-off places. I would think about the future, where I saw nothing but darkness for my son—my lovely little black-eyed boy whom I loved so deeply.

I was fragile from years of coping with the problems that Asperger's syndrome had brought into my family's lives. I lived on the edge, biting my nails and always so thin from a lack of appetite. If someone dropped a cup, I would literally jump and run at full speed toward the sound shouting, "Are you okay? Are you okay?" The kids would look at me, wondering why Mom was so worried. I no longer had the ability to relax. I was riddled with guilt for bringing a child into the world who lived inside of himself. At times, I wondered if I had done something while I was pregnant that had caused him to have this condition, but it does not work that way. According to the textbooks, it's possibly genetic. It seemed sobbing in an empty room was all I could do. The world kept rising up against us—my lovely, innocent son and this broken woman. I was smashed to pieces inside. How I longed just to sink into a deep sleep and be given peace, but the drive to be there for my children was so strong that I would constantly pick myself up, dust myself off, and with all the strength and determination I could muster, push forward in what felt like a never-ending quest to give my son all the help he needed to develop and succeed in life. Even in all my brokenness, my children needed me.

I sought a place for Graham to voice his emotions

Graham was having such a hard time with school that I wanted to provide an extra platform for him to express his emotions, if indeed anyone could actually tap into them. I decided to take him to weekly counseling sessions at a private clinic; it helped a little. He opened up about his feelings of being bullied and a victim. It became clear that even though he had a victim mentality, it was Graham who was doing the provocation. But at least his voice was being heard.

Chapter 8

Welcome to the World of Education and In-Patient Mental Health Units

Third grade

By the third grade, Graham showed signs of being very different from his peers. While his classmates were exploring sports, Graham bowed out entirely. He could not master running and team sports; in fact, he loathed them. He still loved make-believe games and role playing in the schoolyard. Slowly his schoolyard playtime showed signs of isolation outside of a handful of quiet children who were happy to tag along. Graham was so likeable and so full of that essence of youth that he attracted people to him; he just lost their interest whenever he tried to lead them in a game. His peers were surpassing his limited interests of Lego building and online games, and he had little else to offer them. They were growing and developing; Graham appeared to be "stuck" in his playtime development.

    I am grateful to the staff of Graham's elementary school for being so kind, warm, and loving toward my son. They supported him right up until the end of his elementary school years, emailing me, attending meetings at the local health clinic, and even arranging Graham's first home tutor. Their support was incredible. My son never seemed to be able to articulate his feelings or problems, which meant the mounting frustration and pressures he faced were beyond our ability to understand or resolve. Only Graham had the necessary tools to illuminate the problems, and he offered little insight.

Fourth grade

In January, the school principal assembled a report detailing the number of days Graham had missed school. The report served several purposes, but mainly it was a supporting document for the Department of Education, who took parents to court for too many school absences. This fear had always been in the back of my mind. Every time I "failed" to get Graham into the school, I expected and dreaded the correspondence or phone call that was sure to follow.

I had long since lost that happy longing mothers feel as they stand outside the classroom waiting to collect their children from the day's schooling, interacting and chatting about life. This had come to a complete halt for me, as Graham seldom spent a full day in school from second grade on.

The Irish schooling system is split into three terms—September to December, January to March, and April to June. The principal's report told a story of Graham's educational absences:

To whom it may concern:

Below is the total number of days missed by Graham since returning to school.

Term 1:   He missed 11 of 22 days
Term 2:   He Missed 31 of 53 days.
Term 3:   He missed 3 of 3 days.

Some of these days were missed as a result of appointments with medical professionals. In the case of all absences, I was personally contacted by Graham's mother. No unexplained absence has taken place.

Every morning I attempted to get Graham out of the car and into his school—often taking two hours—but too many days he would end up back home with me, having lost his nerve to go in. I would cry my eyes out and make the call to the school secretary yet again. Graham missed forty-five out of seventy-eight school days; Sophie and James had been absent only five days. This gave me comfort.

There was a buzz at the time about court-appearance laws and penalty fees designed to combat school absences. I was terrified of falling victim to these new rules. I lived in fear because I knew many of Graham's absences were not excused with the physician's letter. I wrote to the Educational and Welfare Officer in the Department of Education explaining Graham's Asperger's diagnosis and the problems his teachers and I were facing in getting Graham into school each morning and keeping him there all day. I literally begged them to meet with Graham's principal, his doctor, and me to form a plan of action for Graham's continuing education, but the meeting never took place. It became clear that once again I was on my own. I learned how to fight for my son. I did research, wrote letters, and kept appointments. And I determined never to give up advocating for my son.

Last day of sixth grade

Graham had been coaxed by his teacher to attend the last-day activities to end his elementary school days. He had completed so little of the sixth grade, but his teacher wanted him to graduate with his class. It was a glorious sunny day, and I felt free and light as I walked across the football field to enter the back gate of the school. I was happy that this would be the end of my having to run after him through that mucky field to try to get him into school. No more sitting in the car with him kicking and screaming that he wanted to go home. No more frantic phone calls to come and collect my child as he thrashed about in the classroom and rolled around under tables. The freedom to close the door on this side of my life, and Graham's life, felt so good—even if it was just for a few minutes.

As I entered the gate, one of the moms, whose son had been in Graham's class since kindergarten, was sitting with her face toward the glorious June sunshine. "Hi," I said as I walked toward her. I hadn't seen her in a long time. "Wow, can you believe it? They are actually finishing elementary school today. Haven't the years flown by?" I will never quite forget that encounter. The mother locked eyes with me. She gave me an intense look then simply turned away. I felt my legs wobble. I wanted the ground to open up and swallow me. This woman probably had no idea what I had endured for so many years or what overwhelming relief had flooded over me that day. I'm certain she had reasons for her attitude toward me. Perhaps her son had encountered problems with Graham, and she had built up resentment. Well, she voiced her resentment with her silence. I wanted to pick up Graham and go home as quickly as I could. With my light feeling of freedom having been short lived, I went home and wept. How I longed for a loving spouse to comfort me in times like these. Dignity is a fragile thing indeed.

High school

The local high school was a two-minute walk from our house. It was decided that Graham should have a special needs assistant since he had had one in elementary school. I had several meetings with his school to give a full account of the problems Graham might run into—new routines, new schedules, new classes—just change in general. The preparation took months to complete, and many people put much effort into trying to ensure that Graham's entry and adjustment to secondary school was a successful one.

Not surprisingly, Graham's attendance slipped, and he was eventually withdrawn from every subject. The noise of the machines in the woodwork class overwhelmed him. The subjects that involved discussions also were overwhelming for him. Graham could only cope with fact-based subjects, not ones where he had to give personal opinions. He would challenge teachers in some subjects and be put out of the classroom. Graham was never shy in correcting someone if he knew the facts. This is what made him come across as arrogant, challenging authority, or just trying to make an adult look dumb. But that was not his intention. He just had to give the correct fact if someone was incorrect about it. I felt sorry for him for not having discernment about when to keep quiet and when to challenge. I have no doubt that some people viewed him as downright disrespectful.[3]

Graham was suspended indefinitely, having completed only a few weeks of school. Everyone involved was deeply disappointed that he had run into so many problems in trying to settle into school. I felt like banging my head against a wall. Every type of education I envisioned for him, no matter how well I had prepared in advance, fell short of my hopes and dreams for him. In desperation, I sat down and penned a letter to a local autism society to try and find any glimmer of opportunity for my son.

I learned of a professor who lived locally and was an expert on Asperger's syndrome (AS). I met with him privately for a consultation. I had wanted to utilize this man's expertise to see if he could give any other slant on Asperger's. He was not shocked to hear that Graham had been unsuccessful in coping with mainstream schooling. "Yes, yes, they are often self-learners, absorbing a vast amount of information themselves." (I was always amazed when someone seemed to understand my son.) What a relief to know that what had seemed like a huge problem (school refusal) was actually a normal part of AS! Sometimes these children can cope, but sometimes they don't, and Graham was not coping.

---

[3] Age has eradicated this problem. Now Graham is an adult, and it has become more acceptable for him to correct other adults if they are discussing facts on any subject. He is now their equal, not an arrogant, cheeky, teenage challenger.

An excerpt from the letter he sent to Graham's psychologist states:

> *. . . the history fits Asperger's syndrome DSM-IV from my discussion with the mother.*
>
> *One of the biggest problems she is encountering with Graham at the moment is the moodiness that he has; he seems to be high for a day or two, and then he has lows. Clearly, moodiness is associated with Asperger's syndrome, and there is scientific literature on the use of Fluoxetine with persons with Asperger's. Also, Tegretol, which is a mood stabilizer, crossed my mind. You will obviously be in a better position to see if his moodiness is mainly due to depressive moods rather than Bipolar Disorder.*
>
> *I think that Graham could also benefit from Pragmatic Language Therapy, which is basically Conversational Skills Therapy with peers, and possibly your speech and language therapist might see him for this Pragmatic Therapy. I have given his mother information on a Mind Reading Skills CD also.*
>
> *The kind of therapy persons with Asperger's syndrome seem to benefit from is more a cognitive type that is focusing on the "here and now," helping them to "read" faces, read eyes, and see things from other children's perspective. . . .*

So the fact remained: Graham had Asperger's syndrome, and there were difficulties associated with the condition. That much I would just have to accept and do my best to help him with the struggles, to learn to live within his condition, and to flourish in spite of it.

Again I sat down and penned a letter to a local autism society to see if they could help me find a more suitable school for my son.

Dear Sirs,

Thanks for your reply via email. I want to give you an overview of my son Graham's educational experience to date. I am, to say the least, desperate to know what I'm to do at this stage. Perhaps you can help me.

Graham has been in and out of mainstream education since kindergarten. There are no words to describe the day-to-day problems we encountered in mainstream school. Just getting him into the classroom each day was a monumental task. He didn't start out with an special needs assistant, so whenever he became distressed, I would have to pull him out of school. I was phoned so many times to come and collect my son, more times that I could actually record. Whenever Graham became agitated, he would thrash about in the classroom like a two-year-old, running around squealing then rolling around on the floor in a fetal position. All of this was in front of kids he had been in school with since junior infants. It was awful for him and for them too. His lack of control over his emotions was humiliating and embarrassing.

When Graham was in no condition to cope any longer, I hired a home tutor. Home tutoring began well, but Graham lost interest quickly. It became clear that he could not be taught at home successfully either.

Later I placed Graham back into mainstream primary school with an special needs assistant. In the meantime, I explored some schools for children with Asperger's syndrome, as Graham had been diagnosed with that condition. I visited one of them and liked it, but transportation would have been an issue. I have two other children to get to school at the same time, and Graham was incapable of taking two public buses to school on his own.

Graham was absent a lot from September till January and did not even complete his Christmas exams. (He never completed any type of exams in all his years of education). One day Graham complained of a toothache and said he wanted to go home. He had fixed his mind on going home and tried to climb out the window. He then began to lash out at the teachers and kick their shins. He threw books and other objects around the room. (Turns out, he indeed did have a cavity that was driving him crazy.) Graham was suspended from school for five weeks. The school had hoped the suspension would put pressure on the local health center to meet and discuss a plan of action to get Graham the education he needed.

My gut instinct is that mainstream, even with special needs assistant, is not a viable educational plan for my son. His history of absences, school refusals, and behavioral problems are proof enough that it is not working.

I am beside myself. Graham is a gifted child with above-average intelligence, who is now at home with little hope, it seems, for a bright future. Graham is depressed and bored. He is a self-learner, and he craves mental stimulation.

I have researched, read, and studied the law, and I understand my son's right to an education, but an educational environment where he feels safe and with people who can cater to his way of learning does not seem to exist. I would uproot my entire family and life tomorrow if I thought I could find an education that suited Graham, a place where his mind could be unlocked and where he stood a chance at securing hope for his future.

Can you please help me to help him? He is almost fourteen years old, and the door is rapidly closing for him to secure an education; there has been so little of it over the past nine years.

Get back to me if you think of anything I have missed.

Sincerely,
Tracy Maguire

The psychologist wants Graham to be assessed as an in-patient

Graham's psychologist decided it was worth our while to admit Graham to a local adolescent center that cared for children with mental health problems. They were to assess him fully for three weeks, and then he would attend a small school in the unit so a solution may be found for Graham's ongoing meltdowns.

I had great respect for Graham's doctor. She was naturally warm, attentive, and nurturing. She was invaluable to me during those years when we first thought about medicating Graham and during the hundreds of meltdowns he had. I would call her, almost hysterically, crying and begging for help when Graham's moods and meltdowns escalated. She treated me with such concern and gentleness. She gained my trust deeply. She never judged me, and I could be very open and honest with her about how I felt raising Graham—my fears and worries. I could be truthful about how harrowing and soul destroying it often was to watch one's child attack any object or person in sight and then to have to sit on him and hold him down until the meltdown passed. I learned very early on to divorce myself emotionally from the situation. He was not attacking *me*, his mom; he was in the height of learning to live with the many mounting pressures that came with living within the confines of Asperger's syndrome. I can sit here today with no emotional wounds long after the bruises have passed. Our relationship is strong and healthy. I am grateful that I somehow grasped that tool during those days. It's a healthy weapon against the emotional pain of dealing with the challenges of Asperger's syndrome.

In May, Graham, Sophie, James, and I were invited by my twin sister, Tonya, and her husband, Paschal, to holiday with them, free of charge, in Sitges, Barcelona. I jumped at the opportunity but made it known that I was a little concerned about taking Graham out of his natural environment; a familiar routine is vital for children with Asperger's syndrome. My sister, who was heavily pregnant, assured me that "we" could handle it. They had always been the ones to come to my rescue over the many years of Graham's house trashing. They lived literally around the corner, and I would call them at the first signs of Graham's arms flapping or his voice falling into a motorized monotone. They would drop everything and arrive within a minute, having the procedure down to fine military precision. They would scoop up Sophie and James and take them to their house for safety. Paschal would come back around to assess the situation and on many occasions, this quiet man would help me restrain Graham. We really felt we could cope with this, even on holiday. We were very mistaken.

Graham was heavily medicated at that time. I hated the drugs he had to take; he gained so much weight. He was bloated and the drugs seemed to have little effect other than to dull his personality. He was out of school, suspended, and I was very optimistic that something positive would come of his upcoming in-patient stay. I tried to relax and enjoy the holiday.

Three days into the holiday, very late one evening, Graham suddenly said he wanted to go home. It was 11:00 p.m. When all finally calmed down and the meltdown had ended, we mopped the milk up from the rented apartment, and I knew that it would be years before I took another holiday. Graham hated being away from his home and his familiar hobbies.

Sitting on the beach killing time before our flight home, I remember feeling apprehensive about my son going to stay at the mental health clinic for teenagers, but I was also so optimistic that this would, and must, produce great results—results I had so longed for. I prayed that they would find a suitable school for Graham and teach me how to help him handle his emotional meltdowns.

The in-patient mental health unit for further assessment

In June, I drove the short distance from our house to the in-patient unit. Despite having spent the evening before crying my eyes out, I assured Graham that this was the most normal thing in the world to be doing. I am not sure he had, back then, the capacity to understand what was happening.

Graham was excited as we drove into a large set of gates. I vividly remember that it was a warm, glorious day, and the trees that lined the driveway that swept up to the old Victorian building brought about a feeling of relaxation to ease my heaviness. The receptionist led us to a small waiting room where Graham sat looking at all the toys. Finally, we were called back.

Graham always gave his best to everything he did. He was a little giddy in his presentation and overly talkative with a more childish tone in his voice, which was always an indication that he was nervous. Once again, I gave more details, more history. I had done this so many times that I could have recited everything in my sleep. It wasn't long before the staff asked Graham if he wanted to see his room. That was my cue to leave. My feet felt glued to the carpet. I wanted to hug him so much. Instead, I gave a rather pathetic and squeaky "See you, Son" as I watched the back of his head disappear up the stairs. I turned around, opened the huge, stately door, and ran to the safety of my car.

The drive home took forever. I wondered what other drivers must have thought of this woman with tears flowing down her distressed face, nose running, and sobs shaking her body. Didn't they know that I had just left my son in a psychiatric unit? It was only 9:00 a.m. on a Monday morning. I came home to an empty house. I had gotten so used to Graham being a constant fixture there over the years. I went straight to his bedroom, sat on his bed, and cried my eyes out all over again.

I phoned a few times during that first day and felt a little bit more uplifted when they gave me accounts of him settling well and playing in the game room with the other adolescents who were staying there. He was refusing to eat, and they asked me to give them a list of his favorite foods. Graham's diet had been a constant problem throughout the years. Because of the heightened sense of taste and smell that comes with Asperger's syndrome, he hated certain textures, tastes, and smells. I compiled a list and called them.

At about 2:00 a.m. that morning, I received a phone call. They asked if I could I please come and collect my son. He was banging his head on a door saying over and over again, "I want to go home." Very quickly, Tonya and Paschal were at my house. With many years of experience, Tonya slipped into the house and quietly motioned for me to go so as not to wake Sophie and James. Paschal, without shoes or socks, drove me to the clinic, which now had a haunting look about it as we approached it in the dead of night.

I had expected a huge commotion as I entered, but it was as deadly calm and quiet as it had been early that morning when I had brought Graham into the building for the first time. We were ushered into a larger room.

I wanted to see Graham, and I felt strange that I couldn't just go to him. As the young doctor recounted what had happened, I practically blew up. I was just so shocked and so disappointed. I felt as if no one could "manage" Graham except for me, and I thought how ridiculous this was considering this was a clinic for adolescents with problems. Surely they were trained and equipped to deal with this. Now that things were calm, I was given the choice of either taking Graham home or leaving him there. I was very agitated by this and fiercely frustrated. Graham had come in here, in part, because he had often done this at school. It was a problem we wanted to tackle, and I wanted to be trained on how to handle it correctly. I saw Graham on the closed-caption monitor. Now he was calm, quiet, and rolled up in a ball under the bed in his room, rocking himself. I looked at Paschal and was so grateful for his presence. I was blessed I had the love and support of my family. When they told Graham we were there to take him home, he ran over to us, teary-eyed but smiling. He would remain a day patient of the unit for another four weeks; that suited us both fine.

Excerpt from the final report from the in-patient mental health clinic:

Graham was referred to this Inpatient Unit with a history of behavioral problems associated with his diagnosis of Asperger's syndrome both in school and at home....

Graham is a 14-year-old boy with Asperger's syndrome, ADHD, Hyperkinetic Disorder, and a history of Sleeping Problems associated with Asperger's syndrome. On admission, Graham's mom, Tracy, reported that Graham had never enjoyed school due to increased levels of noise, light, and smell, which resulted in over-stimulation. When distressed, Graham tends to bang his head against the wall, slap out his arms and lash out....

Developmental history shows that Graham's milestones were essentially normal. Graham's interests range between computer games, science fiction programs, and toy soldier strategy games. He has little tolerance for changes to his routine.

Mental State Examination on Admission to Clinic:

On admission, Graham was presented as a neatly dressed, intelligent 14-year-old who seemed anxious at the time of admission. He spoke at length on matters that interested him e.g. Star Wars and computers and was often difficult to interrupt and tangential in speech at times. There is no evidence of depression or psychotic phenomena either in the family or with Graham.

This Is Our Recommendation:

Graham to continue on Concerta 18mg once daily and his height and weight be monitored regularly.... We also recommend that Mom make contact with the three schools mentioned ... and be reviewed by the referral clinic where he [previously attended].

(End of report)

Chapter 9

Alternative Education

Upon his discharge, I was disappointed with the doctor's report. I was expecting him to give me a behavioral plan for Graham. Instead, I left with a prescription and three new schools to research. So I began compiling my letter of inquiry. It was the middle of July, and he should have been entering into his second year of high school in September. Instead, he sat in his bedroom at home.

The longer he was out of school, the more comfortable he became at home, safe and away from the pressures and stresses that accompanied his involvement in daily school life. I worked so hard at trying to source a school, and I was working against the onslaught of negative criticism directed at me about my ability to help my son. All the while, Graham continued to have meltdowns. But somehow, I was sustained. The in-patient facility agreed that he did indeed respond to a smaller classroom setting. That empowered me to find a school that was suitable for my son's education. I sent out a letter to all the schools I found suitable.

Re: Suitable Placement Enquiry

I refer to my son, who is 14 years of age and has a diagnosis of the following conditions:

- *Asperger's Syndrome*
- *Attention Deficit Hyperactivity Disorder*
- *Sleeping Neurosis (ongoing historically)*

He attends the local child and family center and has a full recent assessment from a local adolescent in-patient center in relation to his medication, behavioral problems, mainstream schooling refusal, and tendency to become aggressive when he cannot "process" his emotions correctly (in school and at home).

He has not been attending mainstream school; at present, I am applying for home tutoring, for the second time in his school life, until I can find a more suitable alternative for Graham by way of an educational placement.

It has been confirmed by In-Unit Clinic House, the in-patient unit, that he does indeed respond better to a smaller class setting. Hence, my requirements for him are as follows:

i) *A smaller class setting*
ii) *Staff trained to deal with the behavioral issues of a child with A.S. and ADHD*
iii) *Accredited curriculum fitting for a child of 14 years with an IQ of 115 and one that will be recognized in the workplace for his future*
iv) *Flexible time keeping to facilitate his sleeping problems (note: he is currently on Concerta XL, which counteracts Melatonin, which was prescribed for his inability to sleep; hence, his sleeping problems have returned)*
v) *Transport must be provided if not within short driving distance of our home, as I have two other school-aged children to also transport to school*

I would ask that you let me know if you have a suitable placement available for my son based upon the above criteria.

Thank you so much for your help.

Slowly the responses trickled in. They most certainly had a placement, but . . . The "buts" ranged from them not accepting him because their curriculum was not adequate for his IQ to there not being any transportation available.

Graham was growing very used to being at home full time. The time pressure was overwhelming to help my son. His medication made him groggy, and it dulled his personality, so I requested that he be taken off all medication. I wanted my son back.

With the close of summer, and no school placement in sight, I had the very difficult decision to formally sign documents to take him off the local high school's register. If I did not sign him off the register, I would not be legally free to source another more suitable school for him. This difficult decision meant I was shutting a door for Graham. I thought, *Will we remain in this "land of the lost"? Have I made the right decision?* I tormented myself day and night. I couldn't even feel a faint essence of joy. I felt overwhelmed by the possible life-changing decisions I found myself having to make on behalf of my lovely son.

I even thought about boarding schools but due to financial hardships, this was not an option. I began a distance-learning course but had to drop out prematurely because I couldn't afford it.

Next, I enrolled Graham in summer youth courses; he was accepted immediately. This course was for children who fell into the higher intelligence IQ range. Unfortunately, once again, my financial hardship made it impossible for him to continue.

New home tutor

Having legally signed Graham off the local school register, I could apply for and secure funding for a home tutor for Graham from the Department of Special Education. I hired a home tutor who spent months patiently reading to Graham's feet, which always stuck out from underneath his bedcovers. Her patience and relaxed approach were exactly the nurturing approach that Graham needed after all the years of school pressures. I grew to love having her in the house. She was very dedicated and really liked Graham. She made both Graham and me feel like ordinary people—something we had not felt in a long time. She took responsibility for Graham, and I felt I could relinquish it to her while she was there. While reading to his feet, she would tell me, "It's grand; I know he hears me." And she was right. If he heard a subject that interested him, he would pipe up and tell her facts on it. She was a breath of fresh air for both of us.

Our home tutor would visit us a few years later to tell me that her time with Graham had filled her with such inspiration. When he had shown a love for learning, digested information, and explored a myriad of topics from black holes to atoms, she realized that she had a deep passion for teaching children in this way. She loved bringing their curiosity to life to explore these topics. She ended up teaching full time at a local high school, inspired by my duvet-hiding child. Graham just seemed to inspire people. Without ever leaving his room, his character and who he is as a person touched people. It gave me hope that my son would be of great value to society just by being who he is.

I find Graham's door to the "land of opportunity"!

My search for an ideal education for my son finally came to fruition via a chance phone call. I contacted a volunteer organization called Aspire and, clutching at straws, explained the problems Graham had had in the school system. The home tutor had been a temporary solution; it would not allow him to obtain an actual accredited education because he would still have to take a state exam. They told me there was a pilot program that was looking for one more child in my area for an online schooling system. It was the miracle I needed!

This online school was an avenue of education for my son that surpassed all others. As it turned out, they needed a child who was computer proficient. Graham had that skill. I wanted to sign him up right then! A meeting was booked with the program leader. She would come out to visit Graham and me at home. It was vital that my son *want* to use this educational system; without that, it was futile.

I talked to Graham about it. He did not seem too interested until I said it was an online, computer-based school program where he could work and be a part of an online community. He got excited when he realized they would be installing an Apple computer. He was a wiz at technology.

The program leader and her team sat down in the dining room. I had compiled a full history of Graham's education, special needs assistants, home tutors, letters to and from schools, etc. I wanted this to work so badly. His home tutor had been wonderful, but I knew that no matter what she taught him, he would never be able to sit through formal exams. And no matter how high his IQ or how intelligent he was, without the necessary mandatory academic credentials, Graham would have nothing to show for all the hours any tutor taught him.

The program leader told me she would love to include Graham in the pilot program, but there was a lot of paperwork to be completed, and part of that was having the Educational Welfare Officer provide a referral letter to the online program. Luckily, I had a long-standing relationship established with the officer. I filed all the paperwork, and soon Graham began as a student.

This pilot program was an online learning community offering an alternative to traditional education for young people unable to attend mainstream schooling due to illness, teenage pregnancy, bullying, phobias, traveling issues, reluctance to learn, disaffection, exclusion, etc. Their purpose statement was to re-engage young people in learning, to rebuild confidence, self-esteem, and social skills, and to provide a custom-made pathway into further education and lifelong learning. The children would be appointed a mentor (a teacher), and the students would be called researchers. They would engage in an online, student-based community discussion forum. The program team leaders monitored this daily, and because they had their own secure server, it was a safe environment for children to engage with others in the online community.

When Graham turned eighteen, he had successfully completed many FETAC[4] qualifications under the care and dedication of an online school team, and I dearly respected and admired them for their help with my son. I noticed how his self-esteem and confidence grew during those years. They treated my son with such respect and gave him so much encouragement over his strengths that he came to love engaging with them. He developed friendships with like-minded peers and thrived.

Graham even gained confidence in his passion for drumming, which was fueled by the encouragement he was given by the online school to record his sessions and share them with the community of students online. It was encouragement like this that aided Graham in wanting to take more lessons to polish his talent.

These first students (researchers) who were part of the now solid online school pilot program are now actively involved in running the regular workshops that are set up as part of social interaction for the new children entering the program. This is one of the most successful alternative inclusion educational programs I have ever seen. It may be modeled on an existing proven method of inclusion education for children outside of the system, but I felt that it was the passion and dedication of the staff that made it such a success. They somehow managed to bring school into a piece of hardware, humanize it, and utilize it to reach out to these children. They reached my son, and it was truly the first time he had ever liked school.

This online school may have given my son the perfect home environment where he was safe to learn and gain recognized FETAC qualifications, but it gave him so much more. He regained his dignity and a respite from pressures of

---

[4] FETAC, the Further Education and Training Awards Council, is an accredited, educational qualification given by the Further Educational Body in Ireland.

mainstream schooling that grated on his autistic characteristics. It gave him peers to interact with. It gave him self-esteem and confidence to be the person he was created to be. It helped him to see his strengths. It gave him exactly what some children need—"an accredited school . . . without walls."

Having successfully completed the qualifications for online school, Graham's confidence was soaring. I saw him in a different light. These last few years have been the best of my life. We chat and have coffee together. I have watched him heal and grow with no pressure.

Graham knew that his online schooling would end when he reached eighteen, and he agonized with me over what he wanted to pursue in life. We found a four-year course for Graham to train as an audio engineer. I helped Graham cope with a new routine—a new bus run and a new environment, all of which reminded me that he still had to live with the downside of having Asperger's syndrome. I prayed that he would find the strength to overcome and to pursue his passion in life—his love of music and his brilliance with technology. I knew Graham's confidence and self-worth would bloom to new heights were he to find it in himself to complete this course.

Chapter 10

My Son Turns Eighteen

On the day my firstborn son turned eighteen, we ate at his favorite restaurant—Pizza Hut. We booked a table for eight. Graham, with great kindness in his heart, agonized over whether people would mind not going to a fancier restaurant. He was not aware at how poignant this place would be for so many of the adults there. It was a true reflection of how far my son had come in learning to live with Asperger's syndrome and how closely bonded we all were as a family.

Restoration

My life is slowing being mended, restored. The littlest things bless me, rejuvenate me—the innocent laughter and giggling of my beautiful daughter, having to clean up hot chocolate spills that trail across my living room floor, seeing chargers for technological toys of every kind plugged into every wall socket. And oh, how I love to really listen to my children—not merely to their words, but to fully absorb the fragrant, soft beauty that flows from their simply loving life and living in the moment. How refreshing that is for me. Would I feel this same intensity had I not raised a child with Asperger's syndrome? Would these precious moments mean less to me? Every day brings with it the potential to add another nugget of gold—precious, tender moments—to my cumulative wealth. What a rich woman I am.

I haven't worked in years, and that has cost me financially. But one day I will pay off the mortgage on this house and pass it onto my son. It has always been my desire to make that provision for Graham. One day I will move into all that I am to do in my life as an individual, and each day will bring more healing of my wounds. I will never be restored to the person I was before I had difficulties, but I will be renewed as the person I am now, a very different woman whose heart has been molded by her son with Asperger's syndrome, and I so welcome this new heart.

Final words

Enjoy getting to know your child as an individual. Laugh with him, learn about his hobbies, and let him know you love him unconditionally and are proud of him. I actually got to see that I was very capable of giving unconditional love to a child whose behavior was unlovable. I would have never known my capabilities or character as a mother had my son not had these challenges. It was a huge gift to me.

If you are taking care of an autistic child, don't be afraid to reach out for help. Take any resources offered. Let people nurse you, the caregiver. Listen to their advice. Above all, be honest and real about how you feel. It's okay to feel weary, exhausted, depressed, and in complete and utter despair. That is a part of the journey. It's okay to doubt every little aspect of your mothering at times, but examine your heart. Do what is best for your child.

Chapter 11

Faith Rising

Life's circumstances and experiences can render vulnerability and panic in even the hardiest adult. Some will turn and cling to family, a spouse, or friends. Some will turn to anger, depression, or give up her will to go on. I turned to the place where I found rest—my faith.

Raised a lukewarm Catholic, I marveled at how I had changed from when I was a young child. I was a little plucky five-year-old who would place her hand on her lips in readiness to blow a kiss goodnight to the Lord. I remember so vividly trying to blow the longest kiss. I just remembering feeling that He was so real and that He loved his little cheeky Tracy. It was a childish gesture that still warms my heart to this day.

The first thing I tell people about my faith is that it is real. Being a Christian means spending time seeking the company of the Lord and learning to be in a relationship with Him and others. Cultivating any relationship takes time and so too with faith. Grace is free. It is that undeserved gift where we can turn to our Almighty, loving God and talk to Him. We can cry out to Him for help, seek wisdom and guidance in difficult situations, and just learn to know that faith moves like a simple wind; it is something we cannot see, hold, or contain, but it's very real. Faith not only gives me assurance of eternal life through the free gift of Jesus Christ, but it also gives me a different perspective on my problems. I realize they are temporal, however painful they are at the time. In the often harsh reality of dealing with and living out our difficult days, I had someone to touch and soothe my groaning heart—Jesus.

I grew into my faith, out of a pain so deep and a brokenness so shattered that only something real would have satisfied the conditions of my life. Many people come to know the Lord out of great pain, and when I look back at how all the things I could not control in my life took shape, I say, "Thank You, Lord." These very things moved me to seek God. I have always sensed how close He was to me; He never left me. Because of that, I can stand on a firm foundation. He was the scaffolding that held me up; of that I am very sure. Nearly everyone who "finds God" when he is battered by trauma in his life says the same thing: it was out of a painful experience that he turned to God. Jesus began as my last resort but became the One I would run to in every area of life. He changed my life. I found a place to rest my heart. I regularly spend time talking with and listening to Him.

The more time we spend in the presence of God, the more God enables us to pour our love onto others. Psychologists agree that a human being who experiences unconditional love is better able to love and care for others. Unlike our limited giving to others of ourselves, which can drain a person's emotions or resources, God's giving to us is inexhaustible. Our circumstances may not change overnight, but we can change how we cope with them. I learned that I had to let God break into my pain. I had to learn to let go and just weep and feel His love sweep over me. I am so grateful that I did not turn to alcohol or some other coping mechanism to try to numb the pain. I am grateful that the "crutch" I chose in those days of great blackness and sorrow was Jesus. He was, and always will be, my hope, my companion, and my Savior.

After the throes of Graham's meltdowns, when silence finally rested in the house, I would let the tears flow and cry out to the Lord. There was no soothing music, no stone-clad serenity of a beautiful old church, no caring voice with great preaching or wise advice; there was just me, a woman kneeling alone in the deepest pain, asking a Friend, an Invisible Companion, to show her love and compassion and to help her help her son. It was real; it was raw. There was purity in this coming together of a human with her Creator. I remained like this, on my knees, howling in pain, for six long years—just me and my Lord.

And that is where my faith began. No fanfare, no huge spiritual experience, just a mother consumed by the worry of her beloved son and the brokenness of her life and heart meeting God where He truly is—in our everyday lives no matter where we are. He is not found in the way we handle chalices, in how we express our reverence of Him, in how or where we confess the wrongs of our actions, in how a church operates, or in how we agree on our expression of worship. We can meet God, with all realness, even while kneeling in a puddle of milk, ketchup, and breakfast cereal and crying our eyes out.

I remember one evening when the Lord spoke to the deepest part of my aching gut. He said, "I will sustain you." That sweet, quiet voice was like a bandage for my soul. I forged a relationship with my constant nighttime companion. It was in the years of my isolation, a time that I hated, where my relationship with the Lord grew.

People always ask me if the Lord healed Graham. I don't have a simple answer. My feelings are that God works with us in a variety of ways. What if Graham was healed of AS? Would I want that? My reply came instantly. I am not sure I would know Graham as "Graham" if he was completely healed of AS. I don't know how much the Lord healed Graham, but I do know that my many hours, months, and years of clinging to Him and begging for help on the kitchen floor did not go unnoticed. Graham still does not like smells, but it has gotten easier over the years. His hatred of being touched has long since been resolved. This is the boy who could not be touched for many years. He has learned how to dull out background noises when he travels; he simply takes his earphones and music with him.

I know that the Lord heals in many ways. I do know that crying out to God will never go unnoticed. I know He is deeply moved by our tears of overwhelming sorrow and heartache. Sometimes, there is a God moment for all us in life. It's a moment when we acknowledge the weakness and frailness in our humanity and affirm Him as God; that's the moment we truly become whole. That's where I found the Lord.

If you have not already, I encourage you to seek the Lord. Ask the Lord to reveal Himself to your heart. I know, dear parent, that you, like me, don't have time to waste. You are overwhelmed with everything you have to do to take care of your child. I have been there; I know what it's like. Run to God.

I believe in a God who takes part in our daily lives; He is not just exclusively available for an hour or so in the solitude of a wonderful church building. He is so much more than that.

As important as it is that I give you details of what worked in helping my son, I can't ignore the Divine help I received. This is not a feel-good Christian book of how I found God and didn't have to do anything else. I had a son who needed a great deal of help. Peace often overtook my emotional distress as I cried out for Jesus to help me. I knew I was experiencing the manifestation of the promises written in the Bible.[5] I was living in the realness of the truth of God's Word.

If you are presently caring for a child with emotional difficulties, then I know you need real help, not just soft words to boost your morale. That was how I felt. Often I couldn't see God, but I knew He was there. I couldn't see Asperger's syndrome, but I knew it was there. I couldn't see a future, but I hoped against the odds that it was there!

I will always describe my daily walk with the Lord as "real." In all my weaknesses and in all my failings, I am just me. I get things right sometimes, and other times I mess up horribly. It's practical for all parents or caregivers to balance both of these

---

[5] Psalm 3:4, 50:15; 2 Corinthians 1:4

things. Pray for help *and* pursue practical help. We never know what avenues God will open, so it's important to do all you can with what is available to you. Waiting is very much a part of faith, hope, and trust.

Demographics

How many people suffer with Asperger's syndrome . . . in the US?

Because AS was only recently identified as a diagnosis, a count of the number of individuals affected by this syndrome is still hard to come by. Recent survey results from the National Institute of Child Health and Mental Development estimate that 1 in 500 people (0.2% of the general population) have some form of AS. Some estimates run between 0.36% and .71%. Among people with Asperger's, the prevalence of males to females diagnosed represents a ratio of 4:1. (www.aane.org)
http://www.aane.org/about_asperger_syndrome/asperger_faqs.html

. . . in Ireland?

Autism is a neurological condition in which a child is unable to relate to people and situations. Physically there is nothing wrong with autistic people. Those with Asperger's syndrome generally have a very high IQ but extremely poor social and communication skills.
http://www.irishhealth.com/article.html?id=431

In Ireland, an estimated 10,000 people suffer from the syndrome, with up to seven times as many men affected as women, according to ASPIRE, the Asperger's Syndrome Association of Ireland.
http://www.irishhealth.com/article.html?id=3265

For parents, getting a diagnosis is often their biggest obstacle. The process can take up to ten years and even then, few primary or secondary schools have the staff and resources to deal with the special needs of children and adolescents with Asperger's, the organization says.

www.aspireireland.ie

...worldwide?

Taking the current world population estimate from ibiblio.org, which is 6.9 billion, and using the figures from the best current studies, we can see that 1 in every 116 people have a form of autism, and that Asperger's is 7/8ths of the spectrum, giving us a 1:101 ratio. Applying that ratio to the world population will give us an approximate figure of 68.3 million people with Asperger's syndrome worldwide.

http://wiki.answers.com/Q/How_many_people_have_Asperger's_Syndrome

Asperger's Syndrome[6]

An autism spectrum disorder

Asperger syndrome (AS) is a neurobiological disorder that is part of a group of conditions called **autism spectrum disorders**. The term "autism spectrum" refers to a range of developmental disabilities that includes autism as well as other disorders with similar characteristics.

They are known as spectrum disorders because the symptoms of each can appear in different combinations and in varying degrees of severity: two children with the same diagnosis, though they may share certain patterns of behavior, can exhibit a wide range of skills and abilities.

As a result, general terms such as "low-functioning," "high-functioning," "autistic tendencies," "pervasive developmental disorder," and others are often used to describe children whose behaviors fall within the spectrum. Kids with AS share many of the same symptoms as those with "high-functioning autism."

It's estimated that 2 out of every 10,100 children have the disorder, according to the National Institute of Neurological

---

[6] This information was provided by KidsHealth®, one of the largest resources online for medically reviewed health information written for parents, kids, and teens. For more articles like this, visit KidsHealth.org or TeensHealth.org. © 1995–2012. The Nemours Foundation/KidsHealth®. All rights reserved. Asperger Syndrome, "Brain and Nervous System," Kid's Health
http://kidshealth.org/parent/medical/brain/asperger.html#

Disorders and Stroke. Boys are more than three to four times more likely than girls to be affected by AS. Because milder cases are being identified more frequently, the incidence appears to be increasing. However, like other autism spectrum disorders, AS is often difficult to diagnose and treat.

About Asperger syndrome

The disorder is named after Hans Asperger, a Viennese pediatrician who, in 1944, first described a set of behavior patterns apparent in some of his patients, mostly males. Asperger noticed that although these boys had normal intelligence and language development, they had severely impaired social skills, were unable to communicate effectively with others, and had poor coordination.

According to the Asperger Syndrome Coalition of the United States, the onset of AS may be later than what is typical in autism—or at least it is recognized later. Many kids are diagnosed after age 3, with most diagnosed between the ages of 5 and 9.

AS is characterized by poor social interactions, obsessions, odd speech patterns, and other peculiar mannerisms. Kids with AS often have few facial expressions and have difficulty reading the body language of others; they might engage in obsessive routines and display an unusual sensitivity to sensory stimuli (for example, they may be bothered by a light that no one else notices; they may cover their ears to block out sounds in the environment; or they might prefer to wear clothing made only of a certain material).

Overall, people with AS are capable of functioning in everyday life, but tend to be somewhat socially immature, relate better to adults than peers, and may be seen by others as odd or eccentric.

Other characteristics of AS may include motor delays, clumsiness, limited interests, and peculiar preoccupations. Adults with AS have trouble demonstrating empathy for others, and social interactions continue to be difficult.

Experts say that AS follows a continuous course and usually lasts a lifetime. However, symptoms can wax and wane over time, and early intervention services can be helpful.

Signs and symptoms

Because the symptoms of AS are often hard to differentiate from other behavioral problems, it's best to let a doctor or other health professional evaluate your child's symptoms. It's not uncommon for a child to be diagnosed with attention deficit hyperactivity disorder (ADHD) before a diagnosis of AS is made later.

A child with AS might have these signs and symptoms:

- inappropriate or minimal social interactions
- conversations almost always revolving around self rather than others
- "scripted," "robotic," or repetitive speech
- lack of "common sense"
- problems with reading, math, or writing skills
- obsession with complex topics such as patterns or music
- average to below-average nonverbal cognitive abilities, though verbal cognitive abilities are usually average to above-average
- awkward movements
- odd behaviors or mannerisms

It's important to note that, unlike kids with autism, those with AS might show no delays in language development; they usually have good grammatical skills and an advanced vocabulary at an early age. However, they typically do exhibit a language disorder they might be very literal and have trouble using language in a social context.

Often there are no obvious delays in cognitive development. Although kids with AS can have problems with attention span and organization, and have skills that seem well developed in some areas and lacking in others, they usually have average and sometimes above-average intelligence.

What causes Asperger syndrome?

Researchers and mental health experts are still investigating the causes of autism and AS. Many believe that the pattern of behavior that characterizes AS may have many causes. Research points to the possibility of brain abnormalities as a cause of AS, given that there have been structural and functional differences in specific regions of the brain recognized by using advanced brain imaging.

There seems to be a hereditary component to AS, and research indicates that in some cases AS may be associated with other mental health disorders such as depression and bipolar disorder.

Contrary to the incorrect assumptions some may make about people with the disorder, AS is not caused by emotional deprivation or the way a person has been brought up. Because some of the behaviors exhibited by someone with AS may be seen by others as intentionally rude, many people wrongly assume that AS is the result of bad parenting—it isn't. It's a neurobiological disorder whose causes are not yet fully understood.

Currently, there is no cure for the disorder—kids with AS become adults with AS. But many lead full and happy lives, and the likelihood of achieving this is enhanced with appropriate education, support, and resources.

A Note to Parents

As a mother of a child with Asperger's syndrome, I wanted to share my son's story with you.

I have no other way of reaching out to you, holding your hand, and encouraging you, which is my heart's desire. I can only reach you through the story of my own journey of the many problems, hindrances, failures, and successes in helping my son live out his life and mold his future within the limitations of his condition.

I had no idea I would write this book until my son reached his eighteenth birthday. I suddenly looked at the journey of this young man's life—all the tears I had shed, the pain and distress that we had endured during beginning years—and my heart was touched. How blessed I felt having had the privilege of walking him through so many difficulties. I was overwhelmed and cried a lot on that day. But the tears were not like the tears of pain in his journey; they were tears of gratitude and hope.

My son's journey was not easy. Nothing ever seemed to make a difference with Graham. Medication did not help. Mainstream schooling was ill fitting for him, and his "meltdowns" were a horrendous part of our daily family life. At twelve, Graham ceased all outside education and hopelessness set into my mind and heart. Tears, isolation, and fear crippled me for many years; yet somehow, as a small family of one adult and three children, we got through with the help of my belief in the love of the Lord, my God, and my warm, caring family.

Today, my young man is my constant source of inspiration for my faith.

Today, this young man inspires my love, hope, and passion for reaching out to parents raising children with Asperger's syndrome.

May your child grow into a wonderful, productive young adult.

I pray that hope will spring out of hopelessness.

Tracy M. Maguire

Resources

The Asperger Syndrome Association of Ireland—ASPIRE
www.aspireireland.ie

Autism Society of Middle Tennessee (ASMT)
http://www.tnautism.org/

Autism Today
www.autismtoday.com

Autism Speaks
http://www.autismspeaks.org

Asperger-Syndrome.me.uk
http://www.asperger-syndrome.me.uk/
—website run by loving parents who want to offer help to anyone who needs it

The Global and Regional Asperger Syndrome Partnership, Inc. (GRASP)
www.grasp.org

Online Asperger Syndrome Information and Support—OASIS
www.aspergersyndrome.org

The National Autistic Society—NAS (UK)
www.nas.org.uk

Asperger Foundation (UK)
www.aspergerfoundation.org.uk
—Variety of information relating to AS for adults, teens, and families

Sibling Organization—support information and advice (UK)
www.sibs.org.uk

Asperger's Association of New England
www.aane.org

Footprints Bookshop in Dublin, Ireland
https://www.facebook.com/pages/Footprints-Bookshop-Talbot-Street/160949157276603

And let's not forget:

www.tracymaguire.com, Tracy Maguire's website providing dates of workshops and conferences